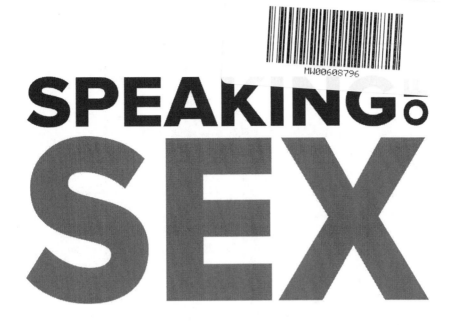

SPEAKING SEX

REIGNITE THE SPARK IN YOUR RELATIONSHIP, SPICE UP YOUR SEX LIFE, AND CREATE LONG-LASTING LOVE.

SHAUNA HARRIS

DOWNLOAD YOUR WORKBOOK *NOW* AS A FREE GIFT TO YOU!

This includes worksheets and fun activities for you to enjoy.

Just to say thanks for buying my book, I would like to give you the Workbook 100% FREE!

TO DOWNLOAD GO TO:

https://exploreintimacy.com/workbook

Dedication

This book is dedicated to my family.

To my husband who taught me that being vulnerable is one of the most courageous gifts that we could give our marriage. I love you so much!

To my kiddos that have taught me how to love unconditionally and have shown me that there is beauty to be found in every situation. It has not only been a pleasure to watch you grow, it has been such an amazing gift to be your momma. I love you from the bottom of my heart!

To my crew that has held my hand, loved me fiercely, and supported me through some pretty extreme adventures. I am beyond grateful for each and every one of you. I love you H, J, M, D, D, C, D, K, K, M, & J!

Contents

Introduction

Sex is such a potent and effective tool to enhance, build, and strengthen your relationship. It is a fantastic way to feel connected and loved and it is a powerful way to show love to your partner. The most satisfying sex lives don't just happen. Sex that is off-the-charts amazing and through-the-roof fantastic *always* starts with a connection. Being emotionally connected with your partner is the difference between "ho hum" and "orgasmic." The more closely connected you feel with your partner, the more you will desire each other and the more you will enjoy having sex. The more you engage in sex with your spouse, the closer you will feel. Of course there is a lot more to dive into here. Women and men respond and think very differently. In order to understand each other sexually, we need to get curious. We need to ask each other questions; we need to learn about each other's bodies and each other's response patterns. The more we know, the more we understand one another. The better we understand one another, the better the outcome will be.

What do you want your sex life to look like? What is your finish line? When you have a finish line in mind, you will know that you have done the work. You will know when you have successfully reached your goal. Create a picture in your mind. What does it look like to have a kick ass sex life? What would your marriage or your relationship look like if your sex life was all that you have wanted and dreamed of? When you have a clear vision of where you want to go, then you can begin to see the exact way in which you are headed. The fog will clear, you will be able to commit to the journey, and you will more easily trust in the process. When you make the decision to put it out there, that you want to improve your life between the sheets, but without a plan or a direction, the tendency is to get lost and frustration arises. More often than not this frustration builds and builds to a point where you want to throw in the towel and give up. Things are not changing the way you had hoped and wanted so you quit trying. But not this time! This time the decision to make some changes and turn things around in your sex life will look different. You will make the decision and commit to the journey but *this time* I will take you down a different path. This path is one that has been proven to increase the passion and the fun in your intimate relationship. This path is not an overnight or a click-your-heels-together solution; it is an ongoing, continuous process that is simple, easy to follow and it works. If you are looking to capitalize on communication skills that will spice up your sex life and add some effective tools to your relationship and sex tool box, this book is for you.

"Sex is...perfectly natural. It's something that's pleasurable. It's enjoyable and it enhances a relationship."

Sue Johanson

Chapter 1

Time For Some Changes

So, you are dissatisfied with your sex life, I get it. We have all been there, or will get there at some point and it can be extremely frustrating. The more we think about it, the worse it seems to get. The more we bring it up with our spouse (if in fact we actually do bring it up with our spouse or partner) the more conflict seems to arise and the more distant we get.

There can be so many different culprits or reasons as to why our sex life has moved its way down your priority list. Please know that you are definitely not alone. Relationships are not easy. They require a lot of teamwork and communication; they are definitely not like the movies as Hollywood depicts them to be. We are pulled in so many different directions the minute our feet hit the floor each morning that it's no wonder our sex life takes a back seat. We have jobs, either inside or outside of the home that require a big chunk of our time and our energy. Our homes need routine upkeep and cleaning. If you have kids, they are a full-time job all by themselves. If they are of a certain age, they require a fulltime car service to all of their sports, recreational, and after school activities. The days are never dull and if there is a lull in the schedule, something is not right or someone in the family is ill. The grocery store needs weekly visits so that your fam can continue to be nourished and fed. There are countless other errands that seem to be on the "To Do List" as well. There are medical appointments, prescriptions to fill or refill, trips to the dry cleaners, bills need to be paid, the car needs gas or routine maintenance, the dog needs to be walked or taken to the vet. Somebody is always needing something from you or needing something to be done.

I almost failed to mention your own social life, if you have any time left for that. You have your girls' nights out or your guy has his regular guys' night, you have your date nights, your extended family phone calls and visits that need care and attention. I am feeling anxious and starting to sweat just writing this out. Of course, every family looks slightly different but the bottom line here is that we are all busy, we all have a million and one things to do every day and it can be overly taxing, anxiety invoking, and very exhausting.

It is interesting to note that when things get tough, when life gets busy, often the first thing to go is our sex life. We tend to focus on the logistics of things that need to be checked off our list, and the emotional aspect of our relationship gets benched. We have to begin to be more aware when we feel ourselves starting to neglect the attempts at connection and intimacy. Connection is crucial for the vitality of our relationship and our sex lives.

What we need to realize is that it doesn't take a huge amount of work to bring our sex life back on track and reignite that fire. You obviously realize that things need to change—that is why you are here—and that is the most difficult step. Congrats, you are well on your way to a mind-blowing, fun, and exciting life between the sheets once again. And, if you have never experienced this type of sex life, you too can now create one that you would be proud to write home about. Or, you might even create one that is so satisfying that you probably shouldn't write home about it.

You first need to simply decide that you are going to have the sex life that you desire. Claim it and in no time it will be yours. Set a goal for yourself and every day you will work towards it. So often, in a session, a client will talk about being committed to attaining the goal of giving their sex lives an overhaul and then they feel completely overwhelmed. In their minds, it seems like such a chore to get to a place that they have envisioned or that they have dreamed about. This is the point where it's time to take a big, deep, cleansing breath and just let those feelings go. It's at this time that we need to simplify the process. This doesn't need to be tedious, nor dreaded. This can and will turn around without blood, sweat, and tears.

So here it is: this is what it looks like without all of the details and the juicy bits. This is how very simple I describe the road ahead: every interaction, every conversation that you have with your partner is either propelling you closer to your goal or further away. It is as bare bones as that. If we can look at it as a staircase that you can start to climb one day at a time, you will reach your goal. If we can just strip it down to the basics, that goal begins to look attainable.

When you look in the rear view mirror at where your relationship started and how it began, what did it look like? For the vast majority of us, it was simple. It consisted of two people who wanted to spend as much time together as they possibly could. It was a couple who brought out the best versions of themselves, who made each other a priority, and who couldn't get enough of each other. This is where we need to go and exactly what we need to remind each other of. You can get that feeling back and it's time to get started.

One thing that we need to be super clear about though, before we really dive deep, is that the staircase doesn't end when your sex life is one of explosive and scintillating fireworks. This staircase doesn't end, *ever*. What I mean by this is that passionate relationships remain this way because two people have decided to maintain the passion. They have decided that they are going to make one another a priority and they are going to make it what they want to make it. There is no half-assing in the game of love and amazing sex. We simply decide that we are going to nurture our relationship and our sex life on a regular basis, and our relationship and our sex life will grow and continue to thrive.

This isn't an "if," it is a "when." This isn't up for negotiation about whether you can re-create those butterflies in your stomach again. It is a matter of you simply deciding, to put in the steps and the work, and then reaping the rewards for years to come. This has been done countless times before and it will happen countless times in the future. When we know better, we do better so let's get some of this knowledge out in the open and watch the sparks begin to fly.

Your sex life is about to embark on a renovation, so let's get this new chapter of your life started. I invite you to enjoy the process and really take the time to be open-minded to the possibilities that this journey has on tap for you. This is *not* a quick fix. With time and effort on your part this process becomes an integral part of your life. You will not look back. You will not regret one minute of it. Allow yourself to have fun with it too. Don't take yourself too seriously. Marriage and long term relationships are entered into with the understanding that there will be many more good days than not so good days. This relationship is meant to stretch you and evolve you. It is meant to be a continued path of learning, together. Your sex life shouldn't be any different. Sex should be fun and enjoyable, so let's commit to giving it all you've got and give yourself and your partner that gift too. It will be more than worth the time and the effort that you invest.

Now, we weren't born knowing about sex and sexual behavior, just like we weren't born knowing how to talk, to walk, or to do long division. It's a learned behavior and because our bodies are so unique, we all have different places that we like to touch and different ones that, if touched, can be a serious turn off. How can we expect our partner to know the ins and outs of our bodies when we don't tell them or we might not even know ourselves?

We jump to conclusions based on what we have heard from friends, seen in movies, read in a book, inferred from a past partner, or copied from watching porn. These are definitely not great resources when applying them to what your partner needs and wants in the bedroom. Go to the source! Only your partner knows that a kiss on a certain spot of their neck is a definite, "It's ON," or that a certain serenaded song in your ear will get you going. You can't get that from a website or a past experience; you must learn that from your partner. And let's get real about erotica, movies, and pornography for a minute. I understand that this is where a lot of the population receives the majority of their very limited sex education and this saddens me somewhat. Why, because this is not reality...let me repeat, this is not reality!

Can you walk away from those resources with a few good nuggets? Of course, you can re-create some fun and interesting positions or scenarios, you can maybe discover certain things that turn you on and entertain you, but please understand that it is not a complete picture of a realistic and healthy sex life. Am I saying stay away? No, of course not but, as a sex educator, I would suggest and highly recommend that you look to your partner as your main source of inspiration. They are your best resource and as you start to uncover the many layers of their sexuality, you will also see more layers that you have yet to discover of your own sexuality. I am going to walk you through just how to do that. We are all sexual beings and it is about time that we gave ourselves permission to be our best sexual selves.

What would your sex life look like if you each gave yourselves the "ok" to just be sexually free with each other, without any fears or insecurities getting in the way? Take a minute and just sit with that thought. Feels good doesn't it? This can be you, this can be your sex life. This will be you, this will be your sex life if you decide it to be!

In the chapters that follow, I am going to show you why communication is so important in the overall satisfaction of your sex life, what healthy communication looks like, how to reach the goal of effective communication, and how to successfully resolve conflict. I will explain the different types of intimacy in a marriage or relationship and why communicating affects each one specifically. I will take you on a unique Seven Day Challenge to help educate you on some pretty exciting benefits of having a little or a lot of sex, depending on your preference.

Please do not forget to grab your *free* workbook that is available at https://www.exploreintimacy.com/workbook. This workbook will help you learn the strategies and tips to incorporate into your relationship. It is a great tool to have on hand as you read your way through this book. Enjoy!

"Lack of communication can ruin the best of intentions."

Shauna Harris

Chapter 2

Communication Is
Where It's At

I've read and heard many times in my life that it takes money to make the world go around. I understand what is being said here, that money is in fact the general medium of exchange but does it make the world go around? I have a different perspective here. If I had to choose a better substitute for what I believe makes the world continue to spin, it would be communication. There is not one single exchange that occurs on this planet successfully without some form of communication.

Communication, when done in an effective and intentional manner, can turn even the darkest of situations into a myriad of colors. Working with couples and learning through my own experiences have opened my eyes to the extreme importance of communication in the long term success of marriages and relationships. Even the strongest and closest of couples will not survive without a continuous effort in the communication department.

Life throws curve balls at a rapid rate of speed sometimes. If we have difficulties in being vulnerable and sharing what is going on in our inner worlds, the foundation that we have been making an effort to build together will crumble and fall. As individuals, we have the intrinsic need to be heard, to be loved, to be supported, to feel safe, and to be accepted.

Committing to a relationship means that making sure these needs are heard and met are a very important part of our job requirements. We have essentially signed on the dotted line to show up for ourself and for our partner. Just as in any other agreement that we make, we do it, we fulfill our promise, no questions asked! Well, that is not actually true in this situation at all. There should be, and definitely needs to be, a never-ending, steady stream of questions between the two of you until the day you are deceased. Do not allow your "Curious George" gene to ever get lazy. Never stop asking questions or being curious about your partner or spouse.

I am going to share with you some tips and strategies that you will be able to use right away. How would it feel to be totally heard and understood by your partner? How would it be for you to feel like you are on the same page with your partner? What would your relationship look like if communication with your spouse or partner wasn't a constant challenge but rather something you both did and both enjoyed together? What if you were able to feel safe to be vulnerable? What would your relationship look like if needs were expressed freely without fear or reluctance? Take a minute to envision what that would and could be for you and the person whom you have chosen to go on this journey called "life" together.

Now that you have a picture in your mind of what things could look like, let's dive in. It is time to expound upon how you can implement a few simple strategies and tips that will actually get you the kind of relationship that you are striving for. You and your partner will be able to use these strategies and tips successfully for the rest of your lives.

Why is Communication So Important?

I would say that the most common reasons clients come to me to work through and resolve in their sex lives are:

1. Communication struggles
2. Mismatched sexual desire
3. "Boring" sex lives

What they don't realize is that all three can be vastly improved with one decision. Do you want to improve your sex life? Obviously, you are reading this book so the intent is clear. When clients come to me, they have decided to seek some guidance but that decision needs more than just an, "Of course I do!" Making the decision is the easy part: you need to commit to the process; you need to be prepared to do the work. Nothing is more frustrating than when people want to make a change but don't put in the work. I am going to give you all of the tools to be successful. You just need to add the intention, effective communication, and the commitment to take the steps to achieve the goal that you and your partner set.

I was in a long term marriage for over eighteen years and so you would think that I would have had my communication game on point. *I did not.* Communication was not a welcome guest at our table. It was done when absolutely necessary and it never was deeply connecting. I was a perfectionist and avoided ruffling feathers; I wanted to make things appear as though they were "good" at all times, even when they weren't.

I sacrificed what was happening inside myself—my feelings, my needs, my dreams for an unrealistic and unattainable goal. When you don't speak out and make this a routine practice in your relationship, the expectation of you not having anything to say becomes the norm. And because feelings are fluid and are ever-changing, this was a ridiculous norm to accept.

A relationship needs to be a safe place to fall, a safe place to be raw and real and unapologetically you, without judgment. Even if there are reservations or uncomfortable spots that make it difficult to open up, these can be worked on and ironed out. Expecting hurdles in our relationship is reality and so if we know what to do when we trip over life or fall flat on our faces, it will be much easier to get up and recover with grace, and hopefully, a little more wisdom going forward. We were created to connect and connecting means sharing and trusting and supporting and accepting one another through our journeys.

Now, years later, I find myself in a completely opposite kind of marriage. It is one where communication is not only the norm, it is expected and expected on the daily. I found this to be such a weird and alternate universe at first. I was super skeptical and often internally questioned my husband's intentions, "Why do you want to know how I am feeling? What do you really want or what are you really after?" Coming from a place of fear, I often asked myself, "Does he have some weird underlying motive? Why is he so interested in what I have to say or what I think all of the time?"

It has been so interesting to me to be in a relationship where communication is expected and encouraged and feelings are shared whenever they come up. This normality was so different and challenging to me at first. I questioned the intention behind the willingness to be so vulnerable. I found it to be so intriguing, yet incredibly overwhelming that someone would be so eager and so honest with what was going on behind the mask. And this wasn't a one-time deal or a short time thing either. I thought it would fade or get old after a period of time too but *nope!* My husband shows up for me every day and is genuinely interested in me and what is going on with me, both in my mind and in my heart. *What?*

I have now come to realize that this, this is what a healthy relationship looks like. I have heard this said and read it many times before and I am not sure exactly who said it but, "You end up with the people who you need, not necessarily the ones you think you need." I didn't think I needed to be held accountable for my vulnerability. Who knew? Something that I steered clear of and hid securely behind a brick wall was one of the most important things that I needed to learn.

Feeling safe to be vulnerable was an Everest for me to climb but my partner was so supportive and so willing to work within my timeline that the walls just continue to crumble. It is so much easier to just let go and express myself. The shared feelings that come along, are so strong and bonding, that they are truly life changing in relationships. Communication builds the trust we need to feel that desired sense of safety to allow ourselves to be vulnerable. I grew up thinking that being vulnerable was such a weakness and who wants to be perceived as weak? Not me, not ever. Through my inner transformation, education, training, and working with couples I now see the people who choose to be vulnerable often have super hero capes draped around their necks or an immense stamp of courage across their chest. It is such an act of courage and bravery to "expose" your innermost self but the payoffs are substantial, transformative, and ongoing.

When you take the time to regularly check in on your spouse, it is much easier to stay on the same page. And when I say on the same page, I mean with everything including, but not limited to, goals, finances, parenting, dates, sex, spirituality, division of household chores, and whatever else may be important to you and/or your partner. It is a whole lot easier to get back on track when you are both intentionally supporting and are really there for one another.

Now, this looks different for every couple for sure. Some like to connect over a morning coffee or breakfast, some like to save it for a chat before bed or nightly walk, others like to plan to check in on a designated night per week. Whatever works for you works for you. This needs to be a priority that is not sidelined, for any reason. It could be ten minutes or it could be for an hour at a time. Again there are no set rules, only just that you do it. It is the difference between a solid foundation or a crumbly one. This is part of the building blocks to your forever relationship: the stronger the foundation, the longer and stronger it will hold up.

When we focus on our relationship and make it a priority, a vast amount of notable things start to happen and continue to occur. When we are able to express ourselves, our partner is made aware of how we are feeling and what our needs are. So many couples I meet assume to know what their partner's needs are and unless these needs have been verbalized and made clear, there is no way the partners can know this with complete accuracy. If needs are not being met in any relationship, trouble is looming on the horizon.

Communicating with our partners fulfills the need that we all have of being heard. Being heard is such a gift that we give, not only to our partners but to anyone with whom we relate. When we listen to hear and to understand, instead of listening to respond, we allow our partners the freedom to express what they have on their mind. While we are actively listening, we are also building trust, giving support, and making them feel safe. We are focusing on them, which is a great act of love, respect, and acceptance.

For comparison's sake, I want to take a few minutes to paint a picture of what ineffective communication is. I know that it may seem incredibly obvious but there are a few characteristics of ineffective communication that I want to illuminate, just so we are more aware. Some of these are incredibly common and many of us do not have a clue that they are habitual aspects of our daily conversations. Although the intention behind these examples may be trying to do the right thing with the right intention, they leave us disconnected. So what does this look like, you may ask? Well, ineffective communication is not an ongoing, steady stream of conversation. It may be day to day, surface level talk but it rarely goes deep to a connecting and vulnerable place. Because of this, topics like sex or meeting each other's needs become emotionally charged or even "off the table" or taboo topics. When there is a disconnect between couples, it is easy for anger and resentment to build because the needs are not being met.

Those who are engaging in ineffective communication also like to listen to fix. I know a lot of you know exactly what these types of conversations look like and end like. The intention behind "listening to fix" is usually good. Our partners are used to solving problems.

The number of thoughts that we typically think on a day is usually somewhere between sixty thousand and seventy thousand. If we take that amount and break it down into the number of problems that we have to deal with and find a solution for, big or small, consciously or unconsciously, we are masters of problem solving. It is somewhat of an automatic reflex, an issue arises, boom we find a solution to it and move on. Well, problems may work like this but relationships do not. We tend to turn on the logical part of our brain when our spouse or partner presents a conundrum and when we see them struggling, we want to jump in, rescue and take the pain away. In theory, this sounds extremely helpful but it is not.

Unless you are asked for your advice and ways to help resolve the issue, your job is to listen. Listening to understand where your partner is coming from is one of the greatest gifts that we can give to them. Showing empathy and compassion breeds a sense of trust, safety, and connection. Many times a shoulder to cry on and an ear to listen are exactly what your partner needs. What it does for the level of connection and the level of intimacy in your relationship is substantial.

Another common word that comes up in sessions is interrupting. Again, your intention might be to help them complete their thought but it is not yours to complete. Let your partner have the freedom to express what they need to say in the time and with the respect that they need to express it. Interrupting each other is disrespectful; it conveys to your spouse that you do not really care what they have to say and that your voice is more important than theirs. These are not good messages to send the one we love, ever.

There are many little things that we do that block or interfere with the flow of conversation but I saved this big fumble for the last. When we get distracted and lose our focus, the trajectory of the conversation changes. Distractions come in a ton of forms all the way from our pets, to kids, to the TV, to work, to social media, to our mass collection of devices. When we choose not to focus on the person in front of us who is trying to express themselves, we are sending a very clear message that they aren't worth our time and what they have to say has little relevance in our life at this moment. This is not the message that we want our spouse to receive and it most certainly isn't what we aim to communicate to them.

The world out there as we know it, in my opinion, doesn't put enough value on the simple act of effectively communicating. When done in a loving and intentional manner, it can spark a fire that was thought to have fizzled. It can re-create those feelings that we all had when we first met and couldn't spend enough time together. Can you remember when you used to rush home to get ready for a date or your heart skipped a beat when their number came up on your screen? Or when something exciting happened and you couldn't wait to tell them? Or your day was the worst and you just couldn't wait to be held and be comforted? Well, it doesn't just have to be a part of your past. It can be like that now. It can be re-created and it can be a part of your relationship again. I have seen it multiple times and it doesn't even take psychosurgery or a strike of lightning to rekindle. It is just simple steps that are routinely executed in your relationship that can turn your marriage from barely there to can't wait to share.

The best way to make the most of these steps and tips is by using them. It all looks good on paper but unless you actually utilize these strategies, they will remain on the page and the communication with your partner will stay one-sided and one dimensional. Everything that I am going to share with you here is super simple and easy to implement. You will need to intentionally keep using these strategies and tips until they become just a part of your daily chats. Any type of change feels weird and uncomfortable at first because it is something new and it doesn't quite feel natural yet. But after a few attempts, along with the proof that you will begin to see in your successful outcomes, they will become automatic. The more you know about your partner, the deeper the understanding that you will have for one another. The deeper your understanding, the less chance for miscommunication. This is why effective communication is the glue that binds. It is the tool that increases the level of intimacy in *every* aspect of your relationship.

We sometimes find ourselves in a place where the communication in our relationships has been or is being taken for granted. We don't treat it as the precious commodity that it is. It has the incredible power to do many positive things in our lives but if we are not careful, it can do extreme damage as well. Communication has the power to hurt, it has the power to divide, it has the power to heal, it has the power to connect and unite, it has the power to turn the worst of situations into something so beautiful and so majestic that it can take your breath away.

This is why intention is so important. So much damage can be done simply with the choice of our words and the way in which we chose to convey them. Words can always be forgiven, yes, but it is often hard to forget them when we have been on the receiving end of some seriously potent interactions. They can leave scars that last for years to come if we allow this part of our relationship to falter. We have ultimately been given a crucial instrument, that if used effectively, can be so extremely valuable in creating the most beautiful relationship that we could ever imagine.

"Communication works for those who work at it."

John Powell

Chapter 3

What Is
Effective Communication?

What does effective communication actually look like if we were to look at it from a bird's eye view? Well, the big picture will look different for every couple but the skeleton of effective communication is generally the same or very similar no matter from which angle. When we walk away or finish a conversation with our spouse and it has gone well, because we typically feel good, we feel somewhat connected and satisfied with the outcome. When a conversation has gone south at some point in an exchange and the end result was nowhere near what we had intended or planned, we are bothered and we feel disconnected. It's not a warm and fuzzy feeling that runs through our veins. We may feel a mix of emotions from anger to sadness or maybe we are left feeling misunderstood or lonely. So many feelings can be bubbling over when things don't go well or don't go as initially planned. If we take the obvious reasons out of the equation and look at the difference between why some conversations go well and some, do not, it usually boils down to a couple of common traits.

When we are continuously sharing information back and forth between ourselves and our partner, while both being active listeners and engaging in the conversation, we are effectively communicating. It occurs in an honest, safe, and trusting environment where both people in the relationship show up and choose to be present.

There are three significant aspects of building a great foundation for an effective conversation in a supportive, trusting, and safe environment. The three aspects are:

- Accessibility
- **Responsiveness**
- Engagement

The assessment that I have included in your workbook is used by many coaches, counselors, and therapists to illustrate the current state of the emotional responsiveness between couples. It is referred to as the A-R-E Assessment in couple's counseling or coaching and in Dr. Sue Johnson's book, *Hold Me Tight* (2008), she introduces and includes the A-R-E questionnaire. The premise of this assessment is divided into 3 sections that ask questions about how **accessible** you are to your partner when they reach out or make an effort to talk to you. Do you avoid certain topics just because they are not important or of interest to you? If they are important to your partner and he/she would like to talk about certain things, they need to be heard; they need to be discussed. Are you **responsive** when your partner does begin a conversation with you? Can you be counted on? Are you there for them? If you can answer "yes" to these questions, you are fostering a healthy and safe environment for effective communication. This makes your partner feel safe to be vulnerable, more confident to share feelings, and more trusting of you with regards to sharing what is important to them.

Do you make an effort to be present and **engage** in conversations with your partner? What does this look like? It means that yes, you need to focus on what your partner is trying to communicate and for you to actually show up. We all need to feel that we are heard, that what we say matters, and that we are important to our partners. I have included a copy of the A-R-E Assessment for you and your partner to take for a spin and see where you both are right now when it comes to your accessibility, responsiveness, and engagement.

This is a useful tool to make you aware of how you are showing up in your partner's eyes and how they are showing up in yours. If you can take this information and learn and grow from it, your relationship can't help but grow and you will be able to communicate more effectively when you are both aware of your strengths and weaknesses. We all have things that we need to work on and we all have things that we kick butt at. Why not give yourself and your marriage or relationship the best chance of successful communication?

This lil' tool can open your eyes to help you see some specific areas that need some work and some areas where you can puff out your chest and be proud. Take the fifteen-question assessment in your workbook as a starting point or a baseline to where you are headed or where you want to go with your partner. Being aware is one of the first steps in the right direction to achieving your goal. Your sex life and the level of intimacy in your relationship is about to begin its evolution. Hang onto each other tight, as this is going to be a fun ride.

When you have finished answering the true/false questions, add up your points. If you scored seven or above, you are well on your way to creating a strong foundation of open and effective communication. If you scored below seven, this is a good time to begin to focus on using the techniques and the tools that are provided in this book to strengthen your connection to build your foundation to forever.

Whatever results you ended up with in the assessment are great. Why are they great, you ask? Well, it gives us a baseline of where you are right now, in this very moment, and that is important information. Do not stress or worry about how you scored because where you and your relationship are headed is not where you are right now. Right now is just the first step to identifying the starting gate. You know where you are right now and you need to accept that for what it is. The exciting part is that you know where you want to be and every step from here on out is going to get you closer to your goal.

We now know how important effective communication is in creating a strong connection in our marriage or relationship but exactly how do we create and execute this type of communication effectively? Some of you may feel like this is where things fall apart because it can be so hard to get through what you actually are trying to convey. You may feel like you hit a wall, you may feel unheard or misunderstood. Instead of placing the blame in any direction, let's take a peek at ourselves and what we are bringing to the conversation right from the get go. Before you even open your mouth to convey a thought, a feeling, an idea, or an opinion, you are saying so much already.

We all are well aware that there are two types of communication in which we convey, verbal and non-verbal, but what we often fail to recognize is the amount of information that is delivered without uttering a single word. We have a breakdown in the relationship coaching world referred to as the 7-38-55 Rule. It is a concept that illustrates the decoding of communication. In 1967, a professor from UCLA, Albert Mehrabian, published his findings on the relative importance of non-verbal and verbal communication. What he found was that the words we choose to use aren't often in alignment with our feelings and our attitudes on the subject at hand. When this happens there is no chance that meaningful and effective communication can happen. Inconsistent messages and miscommunication will undoubtedly result in unfortunate outcomes.

The breakdown of what happens when we engage in a conversation is more than the words we *speak*. It is *how* the words are spoken and it is the *body language* that is occurring during this exchange. The graph below indicates how much we are actually saying without saying a thing.

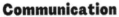

Communication

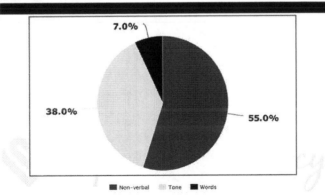

7.0%

38.0%

55.0%

Non-verbal   Tone   Words

Our non-verbal communication and the tone that we use, are so commanding that sometimes the person on the receiving end perceives something very different than what was intended. Non-verbal cues account for approximately 93 percent of what we communicate. This would include tone, body language, and facial expressions. Just think of the looks and the way we contort our face when we are expressing something that we are excited about or have a strong distaste for.

Our entire body, from how we stand, how we hold our arms, if we are leaning in or leaning slightly back, all help to convey a big part of the message that we are sending. Our words account for 7 percent of what is being said, our tone of voice comes in a strong second at 38 percent, and our body language is the clear dominant winner at 55 percent. In order to communicate clearly in the way we would like it to, our words, voice, and body language must be aligned, and supportive of one another in their delivery. This is where things get complicated at times.

I can give you an example that I am sure we all are very familiar with or have heard at some time in a relationship.

Example:

- Verbal: "I am fine!"
- Non-verbal: person looks irritated, avoids eye contact, and has their arms crossed across their chest.

I want to show you how trust plays a vital role in effective communication as well. When your words align with your tone of voice and your body language, there is a feeling of trust that arises. If we look at the example above, the person is clearly not "fine" and therefore not being honest. It might be as simple as he/she just needing a minute before wanting to share what is going on or maybe they do not want to discuss the issue at this time. If this is the case, we align the cues.

- Verbal: "I am feeling a little bit anxious, or annoyed or *insert relevant feeling here,* I don't really want to talk about it right now, I appreciate you checking on me, can we discuss it later?"
- Non-verbal: person looks irritated, avoids eye contact, and has their arms crossed across their chest.

Do you see how the verbal and non-verbal match up here and make sense? This breeds trust and closeness between people. The only thing that we didn't bring up here was tone. So when we respond in a snarky tone, the support of our partner will probably waver so we just need to be aware that the tone we choose matters. If you are feeling snarky, that is okay too but keep in mind how you want the conversation to end. Whatever you put on the table will affect the response and the end result. The bottom line here is that if you have attitudes or feelings to express, make sure that your whole package is on board and calibrated to deliver the message that you intend to send.

Another extremely important aspect of effective communication is your environment. Choosing the best environment for the most effective communication requires some specific ingredients to ensure the highest degree of success. This is not rocket science so don't sweat over the many things to remember, or about getting this right. You will. These things are very much common sense but they do need to be brought up. Sometimes we wonder why a conversation didn't go well when we tried to initiate a discussion about this or that, or maybe it didn't result in our desired outcome and we wonder why. These little details may be the reason. They are tiny but they matter. Let's get into them a little deeper.

Timing — if your two year old is scheduled for a nap in five minutes and your spouse asks to have a chat about something that is bothering him/her that is clearly going to take more than the five minute window, this might not be the best time. If your partner is immersed in Game 7 of the finals, this might not be the best time. If your spouse is prepping for an important presentation or a meeting for work tomorrow, now might not be the best time. You are setting yourself up for a higher chance of a successful chat if the timing works for both of you. This cannot always be planned because things happen, understandably, but there are ways to get around it.

Example:

> "Honey, I know this might not be the best time for a chat but I really would like to talk to you about _insert topic here_. When might be a good time for you to chat?"

Surroundings — are you in a neutral environment? Keep your discussions out of the bedroom and in more of a neutral energy zone. The bedroom, in my opinion, should be kept as your couple zone and reserved for fun, cuddling, and sex. Any other part of the house where it feels comfortable to chat is a great spot to discuss what is on your mind. That could mean inside or even in your backyard. I recommend to some of my clients to go for a walk or a ride in the car, if that is more comfortable for you. Any calming and serene place is a good choice.

Distractions — are there TVs on, playlists running, your dogs are begging for dinner, social media apps open? Are either or both of you in the middle of a video game, or in the middle of a text convo, or trying to multitask? I'm sure you get the point here. No one likes to feel like they aren't a priority. If there is something that is important to your partner, that they would like to discuss, it is important enough to take the time and focus on each other and what needs to be said. Put away the things that tempt you and take you away from your loved one. So much is said here, without even saying a word. When you take the time to show your partner that your attention is one hundred percent centered on them, it breeds connection and successful conversation. At times this is tough. Our minds are going in a million directions, I get it, but if we can retrain ourselves to just stop and shake the distractions for a short time to focus on each other, the course of communication will change and the level of connection will no doubt start to grow.

Privacy — some conversations play out a lot better when there are not little ears listening, friends around, a family of Nosey Nellys nearby, or restaurant staff trying to do their job and unintentionally interrupting. If what's on your mind needs to be shared and it needs some one-on-one time, you need to plan it, create some private time to talk or discuss it. If a discussion is not conducive to the environment, you may not get the results that you were hoping for.

Vulnerability

Do you find it easy to open up and share your vulnerability with your partner? Take a minute to think about it. If you don't, what is it that holds you back?

What keeps you from sharing your innermost feelings? If you were in a position where you felt it was optimal to open up, what would that situation look like? What would that situation feel like? Is there something that you could do to make it easier? Could your partner do something to help you feel at ease or more comfortable with your vulnerability? Here are a few ideas that just might help:

- giving reassurance
- rubbing your back
- holding your hand
- actively listening
- not getting defensive
- hugging
- accepting you as you are
- validating you
- focusing your attention
- not pressuring
- allowing you time to respond in your time
- really hearing you
- making you feel safe
- sitting in the moment
- going for a walk
- going for a drive

It will become a little easier when your partner knows how he/she can help you get to a place where you can become more comfortable with being vulnerable. You can work together as a team. Teamwork is the work that binds and connects. It may not ever become second hat or feel like an automatic shift to the vulnerability zone but it will become a little more comfortable with practice and time.

Being vulnerable, as I mentioned before, was not an easy skill for me to learn. However, communicating with my partner about why it was difficult for me and what would make me feel more comfortable made a world of difference. Coming from an abusive relationship in my first marriage, I needed to feel safe and I needed to feel that I was not rushed or pressured to talk. Now that I realize that I needed those elements in order to be vulnerable, I am able to relay those needs to my husband. Because in my past life I had learned to shut that part of me off as a defense mechanism, and because today my husband is an incredible communicator, we had to find a middle ground. When we needed to resolve a conflict or had something to discuss early on in our relationship, he wanted to resolve the situation *now*. However, because of where I was at, I wanted to want that, but I was incapable of doing it. I would shut down and feel paralyzed by fear. I can vividly remember opening my mouth to speak and nothing would come out. It was frustrating and it was not until I figured out why I shut down and what I needed, that I was able to learn to effectively communicate and be more vulnerable. I know that he needs to resolve issues quickly and I need some time so we compromise and are able to meet in the middle to address both of our needs. Sometimes I still have to catch myself before I go into defensive strategy mode, breathe, and remind myself that I am in a safe place to be vulnerable. Being aware that it has been a pattern for so long makes it easier to have a plan to counteract the trigger and respond in a more productive and effective way.

"During conflict you have two choices; to build a case against the other or to move to understand the other's perspective. If your goal is keeping your love on, then your decision is made."

Danny Silk

Chapter 4

Conflict Resolution -
Put Down The Boxing Gloves

Conflict resolution is a game changer in any relationship. Once the skill is learned, and you have a few experiences under your belt to use it, there is really no disagreement or issue that you cannot solve. It may sound that I am full of smoke here but let me tell you, it works. A few simple steps can defuse any bomb and I can attest to this. I come from a place where I avoided conflict at all costs. In order to keep the peace or not ruffle any feathers, I never brought up my needs or my feelings and for what purpose?

When we choose to avoid conflict and keep feelings and needs inside, we create an environment of distance and distrust, thereby blocking our vulnerability. When we feel we cannot be vulnerable to express our innermost feelings, desires, and dreams, our needs are not met and when push comes to shove, how can these be attained when they are not voiced? What happens when our needs are not met over the years? Trust me, the gap widens.

Communication becomes more challenging when it has been neglected. It needs to be part of your regular routine. How does the saying go? "You lose what you don't use" or "if you don't use it you lose it." It is so true when it comes to talking to your partner. You set a pattern that is hard to break. Feelings, desires, and dreams aren't seen as important when they are in fact, the essence of a relationship. The focus stays pretty one-sided and no relationship will come out alive and successful if it is built on an uneven foundation. Time, care, and attention are the glue to strengthen that base. When that base is constructed with a common goal and worked on together regularly, there is less room for irreparable cracks and damage.

That "uggggh" feeling in the pit of your stomach that may result from a discussion gone wrong or a full-blown fight that came out of the blue, is normal. The presence of conflict in your relationship is not a reflection of whether you and your partner will stay together. Rather, *how* you choose to resolve conflict and *how* you come together during and after conflict is a better indicator. According to psychological researcher and clinician, Dr. John Gottman, the long-term success of a marriage can be predicted by listening to a single conversation. He can analyze a disagreement between a couple and see what conflict resolution pattern they follow. If they make attempts to de-escalate the conflict and their efforts are successful, so too will be their future relationship.

We all have buttons that can be pushed in our relationship or marriage. Things can get messy in a very short amount of time. Again, this is normal, to every healthy union but what I would like to see happen, and I am sure you would agree, is when those buttons are pushed, we can defuse the bomb that could very soon blow the day to smithereens. We usually are aware of what sets us off but where the disconnect comes in is the "what now" spots. In these very crucial spots we have very few seconds to react or to decide to respond.

What I mean by this is that when you are triggered, the sensory information is sent to a part of your brain called the thalamus. Your thalamus then sends the info to the conscious mind or the thinking part of your brain (the neocortex) and then onto the amygdala or the emotional part of your brain. Your amygdala is then responsible for producing the appropriate response. If it senses danger, it will initiate your fight-or-flight response even before your thinking or conscious brain has time to respond. When the body responds to the trigger and you are unable to defuse the bomb, your stress hormones, epinephrine and cortisol, are unleashed. I'm sure everyone knows this feeling well where your heart rate and blood pressure increase, your energy level increases, your pupils dilate, and blood rushes to your brain and your muscles. The body's reaction inhibits you from remaining calm and making the best decisions. Does this help to foster the best environment for effective communication? *Nope!*

Our goal is to become aware of our triggers and become aware of our emotional reactions to our triggers. When we are aware, we can have a plan moving forward to de-escalate ourselves and the situation at hand. If we aren't emotionally aware, our subconscious mind will react with a patterned behavior within seconds, and depending on what our pattern of behavior has been in the past, we know how things usually end. When our stress hormones are released, it only takes 6 seconds for them to dissipate if we can calm ourselves down and not react. However, if we do get worked up and an old pattern takes over, and if we know what to do in this moment, we can turn the freight train around quickly. The sooner the better.

This is where we need to have a plan. When we have a plan and some effective tools in our toolbox, we can make some really positive changes with our spouse or partner in the communication department. Here is where our plan kicks in. Listen up because this has the potential to change your relationship. I say potential because although it works, and works well, it is you and only you who can implement this into your life. So what do we need to do, you ask? Here it is: every time you feel like the blood is beginning to rise like the liquid in a glass thermometer, *stop!*

- Stop what you are doing
- Take a deep breath (preferably 6-7 seconds)
- Identify the trigger
- Continue your slow your breathing
- Ground yourself and bring yourself back to the present moment

When we can become aware of our trigger, slow down your breathing, and feel yourself in the present moment, you are more likely to prevent a reaction and you can thoughtfully prepare a response. As you control your breath, you are calming your central nervous system (CNS) and activating your parasympathetic nervous system (Zaccaro et al., 2018). Your parasympathetic nervous system (PNS) is responsible for activating your rest response and helps you make more constructive and thoughtful decisions. *Ding ding ding!* This is exactly what we need! The human body is so fascinating to me! Some even suggest that a mindful meditation would alleviate the body's reaction to stress (Charoensukmongkol, 2014).

We, as humans, aren't fans of change for the most part. If a behavior that we have exhibited is one of our "go to" responses, the chances of us repeating that behavior are quite high, even if the results aren't positive nor no longer serve us. What we have patterned ourselves to do (probably many, many years ago) is to react, which usually escalates the situation, making it worse. We may get defensive and shut down completely. We may start talking in an attempt to explain, justify, or repair the situation when in fact our actions are making the situation decline faster and further.

When we find ourselves in a heated space without a plan, the outcome is a definite unknown. This generates more feelings of perhaps fear of rejection or fear of abandonment This typically doesn't help to bring the us back together again, nor very successfully. Instead, how about talking about what triggers us outside of the heat, when the climate in the room is neutral? This chat, taking place in a neutral and safe place can help you build a plan of what to do when the next fuse is ignited. When we are triggered, it is hard to be an effective communicator, especially if we are at a loss of what to do next. So, if there is a plan in place that was collectively constructed by the two of you, things are going to start looking a lot different for the two of you going forward.

In your workbook, you will find an exercise that will shine a light on your triggers. We all have them so this is not meant to be a negative experience at all. It is meant to help you be aware of the things that push your buttons and initiate a reaction out of you. When you take the time to discuss why you are triggered when a certain behavior is exhibited or a certain phrase is vocalized, it gives your partner the opportunity to understand why you react the way you do. I can give you

a few examples here to help show exactly how powerful this exercise can be in developing a plan. When we
have the tools to respond, instead of reacting to any
given situation, our level of intimacy grows. When we
react to an event, our emotions often take over and the
situation escalates. Conflict usually ensues after a reaction occurs and the level of intimacy is threatened
or worsened. When we have a plan of how we could
respond when we are triggered, and a plan of some
possible things that we can say, we can set ourselves
up as individuals as a united front for success. When
we take a pause or a deep breath, we are allowing our
nervous system to take a different path than what our
bodies have been used to taking. We can break the patterns that have been ingrained and that have been set
on automatic. We can consciously decide and be aware
of our reactions and switch them into new responsive
patterns.

Example #1:

> You are annoyed that your spouse is looking at their
> phone while you are eating dinner and trying to en-
> gage in a conversation.
>
> **You:** "Can you put your phone down for ten minutes
> so we can talk and enjoy our dinner?"

This will probably not go over too well and invoke a
defensive reaction.

> **Your spouse:** "I am enjoying my dinner, you weren't
> saying anything anyway."

Things may then begin to spiral and get messy. Let's
change up the delivery and see how it could go differently.

> **You:** "Hey honey, I am feeling a little bit disconnected
> from you right now. I would love to talk and spend
> some real time together because I really love feeling

close to you, spending time with you, and hearing about your day. What would you think if we started a no phone policy while we are having dinner. You are important to me and our marriage is important to me."

Example #2:

Your partner has been super busy at work, very distracted, and distant. You feel shut out, left out, sad, and lonely.

You: "Why can't we go out on a date night and have some fun like everyone else that we know?"

Spouse: "Are you kidding me? I have been slammed at work and barely have time to think and you are complaining because we haven't had a date night in a few weeks? Give me a break!"

Again, the delivery here is definitely getting a point across but if it was softened slightly the results would be much more positive and very different.

You: "I know that you have been super busy at work lately and I can understand that. I want you to know that I appreciate you working so hard for our family, I would love to plan some "us" time so that we can have some fun together, what would you think of a date night next week? I have been feeling disconnected and lonely, I miss you.

We can't control how our partner will respond or react but what we can control and focus on is our attitude, and our effort in doing our best to communicate in a clear, concise and effective manner. When you approach your partner in a way that encourages them to turn toward you and be open and willing to meet your needs, your relationship and level of intimacy will completely change. With this approach, you are able to express your feelings as well as create a loving and safe environment. The key here is to lead with your feelings. Why do we want to do this? Well, when you are vulnerable with your partner and begin conversations that are not accusatory, the defensive reaction is less likely to present itself.

We can also control the use of a well-timed and sincere apology. The power of this little beauty is seriously underrated. I didn't realize the potency and the weight that a simple, "I'm sorry" holds until my second marriage. I don't remember hearing those words very much at all until then. It wasn't a phrase that was typically used in a sincere way, so the power of it was lost on me until I learned otherwise. We all mess up therefore, we all need to apologize. The power that is packed into that little phrase isn't just the words though, it is the actions that follow. If we apologize for a behavior that continues and there is little effort to change, the apology loses its validity and creates a breach in trust. I do understand that changing behavior is a process sometimes and it needs time and effort but if there is integrity, intention, and a genuine effort to change then there will be change.

Emotions

When you are trying to connect with your partner, it is crucial that you lead with relevant emotions. Yes, you may be feeling frustrated, disappointed, even resentful but if you were to dig deep into those emotions and look behind them you would find the core emotions, or the root of what is coming up for you. Emotions can be divided into two categories:

1. Primary
2. Secondary

Primary emotions are instinctive, whereas secondary emotions are more intense, usually longer-lasting and come right from the heart. We tend to see and feel the primary emotions first and run with that feeling. If we take the time to examine this, we can really understand what is under those initial fiery feelings. When anger rears its head for instance, yes, we are mad. We might even be furious, but if we can take a breath and sit with that anger for a minute, we will come to understand that the anger really is something more.

When we get into this habit of being responsive, as opposed to reactive, our communication skills become a lot more connecting and effective. So, we initially feel angry but after some self-reflection, we come to realize that we really feel disappointment, rejection, and maybe just downright loneliness. These are emotions that foster compassion and vulnerability in the very ones that we are trying to connect with. Some refer to primary emotions as surface emotions because it is what is seen on the surface, whereas secondary emotions are found at a deeper level. Take a look at the chart below.

PRIMARY EMOTIONS

anger	fear	sadness	joy	love

SECONDARY EMOTIONS

frustration	happiness	vulnerability	shame
disappointment	shame	satisfaction	pride
guilt	optimism	trust	depression
enthusiasm	jealousy	hope	peace
depression	confusion	regret	lonely
pride	anxiety	confidence	satisfaction

Sometimes the visualization of an iceberg works to illustrate this as well. Take a look at the photo here. What you see above the surface isn't the entire picture. There is always a whole lot more going on under the surface and if we aren't careful navigating around the iceberg, we might end up running into it. If we react to a primary emotion, it is very likely going to be a defense strategy that we will grab to combat the situation and protect ourselves. If we are approached with a secondary emotion, the tendency to show up with compassion, understanding, and kindness is a lot more probable. As with all icebergs and emotions, there is so much more than what we initially see. When we take the time to uncover what is beneath the surface, then and only then can we understand what the real issue is and where it is or might be coming from.

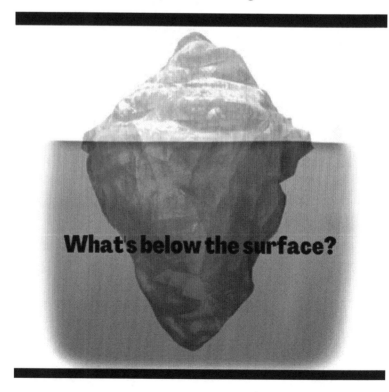

What's below the surface?

To sum this up and make sure we are all on the same page here, when we react, know that we are coming from our survival mode. It's fight-or-flight time and we might regret some of the actions we take or the words that we say. When we stop and breathe and allow ourselves a little more time to respond, we are coming from a more well-thought out place, our conscious mind. Goleman (1995) refers to this as emotional intelligence.

We have been programmed since we were born to do things a certain way and chances are we haven't changed much since our early years. The way we brush our teeth, the way we go through your morning routine, the way we tie our shoes, eat a sandwich, or the way we prepare our coffee or tea. We are very programmed individuals who thrive on routine. Even when those routines aren't working for us anymore we tend to fall back into the same patterns. Guess what? What isn't working for us needs to change. The sex life that has fallen into a rut or has become routine, needs to be switched up. What needs to change is the way we communicate with our partner. It isn't getting us where we want to be, and isn't resulting in the outcome that we want. You can do this by incorporating the changes above that I mentioned in your communication pattern and you can also do this by getting into the habit of using your conscious mind as opposed to your subconscious mind.

When we are in autopilot mode, we are using our subconscious mind. Have you ever pulled into the driveway and thought, I don't even know how I got home? I am sure we all have. It is just habitual, we have done it so many times that, it comes naturally. We need to snap ourselves out of our patterned behaviors to move to the new path. Our routine ways and techniques are incredibly helpful...until they no longer serve us! This is the time for an upgrade. It is no different when it comes to what is going on in our relationship and the way in which we connect with our partner. We are ever-changing as individuals and as a couple so, what worked for you two months, two years, or twenty years ago might not be what is most effective anymore. That is okay. What is not okay is to keep trying the same old techniques and expecting different results.

I learned valuable ways to effectively communicate in my years of training for sure but it was simplified and more clear when I heard it in a course that I took on communication from LMFT, Sam Tielemans. Tielemans stated it so simply, so beautifully, that it was like a light bulb moment for me. The super "user friendly" technique is one that I now implement, to teach my clients, and to use in my marriage. Thank you Sam.

Plain and simply put here is your new effective communication plan:

Partner A:

1. Share how you are feeling
2. Ask for what you need

When you share how you are feeling in a vulnerable way, I encourage you to take some time to look below the surface. Voice those secondary emotions that really get to the root of things and that are important to communicate. When you are expressing yourself, remember that your tone and non-verbal communication should be a match so that you don't confuse your partner. Be careful not to use an accusatory or blaming tone or attitude when you are relaying your message. Your intention needs to be clear.

Partner B:

1. Hear what your partner is communicating
2. Accept and validate your partner
3. Offer comfort

We discussed already how important it is to really hear what our spouse is saying. We all want and need to be heard. Acknowledging what is being said is crucial because it lets our partner know that we are aware of what was said, that what they say is important to us, and the message is relevant. When you connect as a couple *first* and then problem solve, the results will be more on-track with where you want to be. They will be much more effective. When we feel connected, it is much easier to feel calm and not as easy to have our buttons pushed or to be agitated. We all have the ability to regulate our nervous system when we are connected. It is a completely different experience to communicate like this and it will feel completely different, but in a positive way. Sharing how you feel and what you need in this way stimulates a compassionate and a connective response. When more of your needs begin to be met, the easier these steps will become and the connection between the two of you will continue to grow.

Relationships don't end because of a presence of, or an increase in, conflict in a relationship at all. They end as a result of a decrease in connection. I have heard a few times that the opposite of love is not hate, it is indifference. I couldn't agree more. When there is a lack of interest or concern, there are problems on the horizon. So, before you get to that space or even close to it, there are many things that can be done to keep the passion alive or ignite that spark again.

Expecting that conflict will not be a part of your marriage or relationship is not realistic; conflict is actually a very healthy part of your growth and the actual state of your relationship. If you, as a couple, never disagree or never have an argument it should be a red flag. How can two completely different people from two very different paths and life experiences always agree and see things the same way? It is just not possible.

I used to pride myself on the fact that in the first fifteen years of my first marriage, I could probably count the amount of times that we fought on one hand. I am not sure what my thought process was but I am sure the fear of not having things work out (like in my parents' relationship) had something to do with it. I thought that if we didn't fight, we would last forever. I was young. I was naïve, and I didn't know any better. Seeing life through a more mature lens and now having the chance to create a healthy marriage, make things look a lot different these days. Conflict can be a chance to grow together as a couple, as long as you are resolving your conflict in a productive and connecting way. I will show you how to use this connecting conflict resolution technique below.

It's really all about looking at things with a unique perspective and using a different approach.

> *"The definition of insanity is doing the same thing over and over again, but expecting different results."*

I love this quote by Albert Einstein because it rings so true. We get into the habit of doing the same thing over and over yet we expect a different outcome. This makes absolutely no sense and new results will not emerge. We need to try something different to get the desired result if the techniques that we have been using no longer work. It can feel hopeless and frustrating though when we don't know what to do or do not have the tools to try a different approach.

In my current relationship, if something isn't working for one of us, it is brought to the table in a timely manner that is respectful and kind. It is not a one-sided conversation. Each person has the opportunity to voice their feelings and opinions about the topic at hand. If the stream of communication is faltering, it is addressed and we can usually defuse the situation in a manner that leaves both of us feeling heard, supported, and loved. We both still get triggered for sure but we have learned how to navigate conflict in a positive and productive way. Emotionally charged topics are way easier to discuss and become less electric. The more comfortable we become with this process and each other, the more proficient we become at conflict resolution. Here is the process that I now use in my marriage and that I have helped many clients incorporate into their lives. It works. It has been adapted from Sam Tielemans, LMFT (2020), and it has proven to be so incredibly useful. It is simple, it is easy to remember, even in the heat of the moment. This approach instantly changes the energy in the room and fosters a safe environment to be vulnerable.

How to resolve any conflict:

1. **Be aware** of the trigger — what caused the reaction
2. **Clarify**— this is how I'm taking it (taking it personally or misinterpreting)
3. **Validate** your partners feelings

When one of our hot spots or buttons has been pushed, we need to take a moment and be aware of the trigger. What has caused this reaction? What was said? What just happened that triggered me in this way? Once we are aware, we can respond accordingly. I know that this has caused me to want to react in a certain way but I'm going to take a step back, breathe, and think about how I am perceiving what just happened. Am I taking it personally or misinterpreting what he/she has said or done? My best option here is to clarify, so that I am not reacting. When we clarify, we can say something like, "I am not sure what you meant by that, can you please explain it to me a little further?" Or, you could ask, "This is what I just heard, is that what you meant by that?" "I just want to make sure that I heard you correctly, is this what you just said?"

When we get into the habit of clarifying *before* we react, the amount of verbal sparring sessions that will result will be drastically reduced. Why? Because before we react with a potentially inaccurate perception of what was intended, we can give our partner the opportunity to explain what was meant. We are coming from two completely different head spaces and the chance that we may miscommunicate or misinterpret what was intended in the first place is actually pretty high.

Being an effective communicator means taking accountability for what we are saying and how we are being heard. The way we talk about and deliver our message is so important, as it can alter the interpretation of the information that we are trying to communicate. We are surprised and sometimes confused as to why our spouse or partner didn't hear what we "clearly" said. It seems so coherent, so obvious to us when in fact, it may be the exact opposite. Depending on the filter that your partner is listening with at the time, many different things could be heard. Filters are extremely powerful. They distort what is actually being said and we all have them. Are we being sarcastic? Do we have an edge to our tone? Are we being completely honest? Are we being condescending or respectful? Are we conscious of our body language? All of these things play a part in whether we are coming across as we intended and not being misinterpreted. Remember the words that we choose are incredibly important but they are just part of the package that we are delivering to our partner.

Sometimes arguments are brewed from the most unlikely situations and it rarely is about the "thing" that you are heated about. It can start anywhere and can be triggered by the most unexpected event or words. It doesn't just pertain to heated discussions or arguments either. It occurs in everyday easy breezy conversations. Just last night my hubby and I were talking about a show that he really enjoyed. It was a show that I watched with him and although I did find some entertainment in it, it wasn't for the reasons that he thought. It is a silly example but it does illustrate that in any interaction, there are filters.

Example:

> **Hubby**: "You really liked that show and how unpredictable and terrifying it was, just like I did. I also liked watching it with you and making you feel safe."

> **Me** (*in my head*): Ummm, no, that's not why I liked it at all! How I took it was way different than what he intended. First of all, I misinterpreted his comments to mean that I was weak and needed him to watch the show with me, which is hilarious when I took the time to think about it. Knowing him as well as I do, it

was definitely not what he meant. Second of all, I am not like you in this regard at all, as I do not like dark, scary shows.

Me: "I actually don't enjoy being terrified at all and so that is not why I liked the show, I liked the show because the kids were awesome and they worked together to survive."

Me: I laughed at myself and then said to him, "Do you want to know what I heard you just say? I heard you telling me what I liked about the show instead of asking me why I liked the show, which pushed a button. It is interesting to me that I get triggered when I feel my opinion is made for me, it feels like I am being bossed and that my actual opinion doesn't matter, and that makes me feel weak."

We both started to laugh and he grabbed me and hugged me.

Hubby: "You know that I would never even attempt to boss you, I know better. And, that is not what I intended at all. I was just thinking about how much I like to snuggle while we watch a show and I like making you feel safe."

So instead of fighting about how he made me feel, we ended up laughing about it because I was willing to talk about it so that he could clarify what he meant. It turned out he wasn't even really talking about why I liked the show. He was trying to tell me that he liked watching the show with me because it made him feel connected and close. Well, if he just said it that way from the get go, I wouldn't have had my nose in a knot for a minute. Do you see how things could have gone so differently if I had not clarified his intention? It would not have ended in us laughing and embracing and feeling even more connected so soon. We defused the bomb that could have very well blown and it ended with us feeling more connected and not having had fought at all. We actually laughed about it for a few days and it makes me smile to think back on it even now.

Another lesson that has hit home for me in my second marriage and that has been so helpful in my coaching practice is to give your spouse the benefit of the doubt in every situation. Most people's intentions are good. You are both on the same team and so when you think about that, really think about it, your partner wants the best for you and is your biggest supporter. When you feel like you are on the same team, life in general becomes so much easier. How do you get on the same team again? By leaning towards your partner and making intentional efforts to connect on a daily basis. There are and will be days where you are not aligned and that is to be expected but this is also a time to communicate and figure out what needs are not being met and how to get back on track.

Assumptions

When we come to the table with suspicion and assumptions, we are already behind the eight ball, so to speak. Assumptions and expectations are complete relationship killers and need to be kept in check. Assumptions get us nowhere and quickly too. Assuming what your spouse needs or how they feel is like sneezing into the wind. It may initially feel right but it will come back and hit you in the face and then you are left with an, "I may not have made the best choice there," kind of feeling. When we assume the worst, we shut down, our attempts at connecting falter, and we stop making an effort.

What does this bring to the relationship? It brings a lack of trust. It takes away our feeling of safety, and our vulnerability becomes guarded behind a defensive wall. Being aware of your thoughts is the first step and when you feel yourself making assumptions, take a deep breath and take a moment. What do I know to be the truth? Did I actually witness it myself? It is not healthy for your relationship to write your own script. The mind racing needs to slow down and some clarification (as mentioned above) needs to occur.

Trying to read someone's mind is about as productive as running the wrong way up an escalator. Focus on the facts. When you focus on what you know, a more positive solution is inevitable. Do the facts support your beliefs? You may feel strongly about something and don't get me wrong, all feelings are very valid but not all feelings may be accurate either. Stick to what you know to be true; stick to the facts.

When our minds start to spin and we get wound up, it can be easy to look in the rear view mirror. This isn't helpful either. We should stay in the moment, stay in the present, not the past. Just because something painful happened in our past doesn't mean that we need to place ourselves on repeat, so don't let your past lead you into a negative pattern. Keep looking forward and train your brain to think the best. If you take a moment and weigh the cost and benefit of assuming the worst and trying to fill in the gaps, you will soon realize that there is far more to lose when you decide to assume.

When we lead with positive thoughts, they breed more positivity. When we choose to see the good in our partner, we will soon begin to notice that there is more good to be seen. When we take out the action of assuming from the equation, it also has a positive effect on the level of trust in your marriage or relationship. When we are able to create a foundation of trust, the tendency to make assumptions won't be so tempting and we will be reassured by the trust that we have in our relationship and in our partner. When that trust is backed with clarifying questions and effective communication, it is a winning combination.

This also rings true when (a) you are trying to tell your partner about an event that occurred that you are not happy about and (b) all they do is offer you solutions to "fix it." We discussed Mr. or Ms. Fix It already and we have concluded that this is counterproductive, unless you have been specifically asked for possible solutions. Most of the time we just need and want to vent, "spill our guts," and feel heard. We are not asking our spouse to be logical; we need compassion and comfort. We can all understand the intention behind their suggestions and potential solutions, they want to help. They do not like seeing someone that they love upset or suffer, so their first instinct is to fix what is broken or eliminate what is causing the problem.

I know that I have done this with my kiddos too and I wish that I had known better sooner. It is painful when the ones who you love go through tough situations. My instinct was to want to take the pain away as soon as I possibly could but what I failed to do was meet them where they were at. If we can walk away from failure having learned something, it has served its purpose and we can go forward with the new knowledge and be a better version of ourselves. When we ask our loved ones what they need and allow them to express them, we can meet them where they are at and try to give them what they need, and not what we think they need.

An important point that I want to make when discussing conflict and conflict resolution is the use of absolutes. I am sure that we have all heard this before and it does make a lot of sense but it is worth repeating. I am referring here to words and phrases such as:

- Always
- Never
- You are exaggerating
- That is not how it happened
- Why don't you ever…
- You do this every time

These will no doubt elicit a defensive response and will not get you the results that you are looking for. Instead, try in incorporate words and phrases that verify, clarify, and help you reach an outcome that brings the two of you closer, not further apart. Here are a few examples:

- I hear what you are saying…
- I want to understand what you are trying to say, could you please tell me a little bit more.
- Could you please tell me another example of when I made you feel this way so I can be more aware and try not to do it again?
- I can see how you felt like that, can you tell me more about…

If we take away all of the details of each conflict that we have with our spouse or partner and really strip it down to the bare bones, do you know what we would find every single time? An unmet need. You read that right, an *unmet need*. It isn't about the lack of helping around the house, the long hours at work, or the never-ending football games, or long talks with friends on the phone. These are what triggers the unmet needs and when an unmet need is triggered, an argument or a conflict may ensue.

We need to be aware of what caused us to react, or the trigger, and then talk about it. Let's take the example that I hear a lot when clients come to me.

Example:

    Client: "She/he never wants to have sex."

Ok, so if we dissect this gem a little further, there is a lot more going on here than meets the eye. The trigger here is that sex is not occurring as often as the client would like. When this occurs, it is commonly perceived that, "I am no longer desirable or sexy to my partner." The emotions that bubble and expose themselves now could be anger, sadness, loneliness, and/or rejection. This then prompts a reaction. Depending on what the patterned defensive strategy is or the "go to" reaction is, a shutdown occurs. The wall goes up or the defensive battle may begin.

Trigger →	Perception →	Emotion →	Reaction
sex is not happening as often as I want it to	I'm not desirable	anger rejection	shut down defensive

When we can break it down like this chart above, that has been adapted from Sam Tielemans (2020), it is easier to see what causes the reaction and how we can interject or break the cycle. When we have been triggered, we need to stop, take a breath and bring awareness to the moment. What just happened and why am I triggered? It is definitely not as surface level as, "I'm not getting sex 5x/week." I now know and am aware that it is a need that is not being met. "What need do I have that is not being met?" The way I take the rejection is that I am not desirable and my partner doesn't want to have sex with me but logically, I know that is not the case. It makes me feel sad and I get angry. I don't want that because I know that when I feel this way I react. When I react, the result is nowhere near what I had hoped or planned for. When we bring awareness to the situation, the pattern can be broken and new patterns that involve effective communication can be formed. What is the need that is not being met? The unmet need here is connection. I feel close when we are intimate and I need to feel close to you. A conversation could go something like this example below.

Example:

> "Hey Hon, I am feeling a little rejected tonight and instead of me getting angry and defensive, I was wondering if you had a couple of minutes to talk about it?"

> "I love the feeling of being connected and I am feeling really disconnected right now. The easiest way for me to feel connected to you is when we have sex. I know that there are other ways that I can feel close to you but sex is an important part of our relationship to me and I am trying to feel connected to you."

This delivery will go over far better than any defensive reaction or shut down ever will. You could even have a further discussion about other ways that you both could come up with that would meet the need to feel connected and close. Would a bath together be an option or an intimate walk? How about a cuddle fest or a mini make out session? It's always a good idea to have a few options in your back pocket that can help you try and meet the need.

When needs are expressed, then and only then can they be met. If we don't voice what we need, how on earth can we feel truly fulfilled? If you don't bring unmet needs to the table and aren't willing to work through things, your relationship will not grow and will not thrive. Sweeping things under the carpet doesn't work well for too long. Those piles of unresolved issues will keep building and piling up until they are unmanageable and you have no idea how to tackle the mountain that you have created.

Being Triggered

When an emotion comes up for you and you are triggered, it is essentially a message that your body is sending you. If you listen and can sit with the emotion for a few moments, ask yourself, "What can I learn from this? How can I grow from this?" Your body is trying to work out a certain emotion that it no longer wants to hold on to, that no longer serves you. The message you are being sent is that it's time to let me go-it is no longer needed. Take this message as an opportunity to rid yourself of this emotion. This is precisely why we need to work through these triggers and not push them down deeper. When we work through an emotion that seems to be a recurring trigger, we are able to release the grip that it has on us and eventually let it go. We all have triggers and we all are going to be challenged somewhat when they come up. If we can alter our perspective and see these triggered responses as a learning experience and a chance to grow, it will stretch us and help us to heal from past events and traumas that have occurred in our lives. When we can learn to sit comfortably with what comes up for us, we are able to sit alongside another with theirs. Do you see how this can be such an essential tool for our relationship toolbox? The more understanding we can be of ourselves, the more compassionate and understanding we can be to others. This is a definite win-win, in more ways than one.

Your mind is such a powerful tool but you and only you have the power to control your thoughts, your emotions, your responses, your reactions, and your beliefs. What you do with these can set the tone, the stage, and the course of the future of your relationship. Please realize that it takes only one person to change the course of any conversation. We all like to be "right" but if you are given the opportunity to feel connected and closer to your partner or to continue to ignite and fuel, increase the tension and feel disconnected, I know which option I would choose. Being "right" isn't always the best target. If you are aiming for a strong and resilient relationship that will endure the roughest of times and then enjoy the happiest of moments and everything in between, the way you deal with and come together during and after conflict is a huge determining factor.

I have included a page in your workbook that allows you to write down some things that trigger you. Don't overthink it. Triggers are so different for everyone and so there is nothing too "out there." This is just to bring them to light, to make you aware of them. When you are both aware of your triggers, you and your partner can talk about them and be more prepared the next time for an effective response rather than a reaction. If you can start a discussion on what pushes your buttons and the reasons behind it, it helps your partner to be more compassionate and more understanding. When triggers are discussed outside of the "heat of the moment," you and your partner can make a plan that works for both of you. A quick example of this scenario might be when one of you gets triggered, your response might be to recoil and shut down if the discussion begins to escalate. Your partner might take this as rejection and not back down to try and get you to engage in the conversation. These two reactions do not mix well but if you have discussed it beforehand and you have come up with a plan, the discussion can be defused a lot quicker and a lot easier.

Example:

Partner 1:

> "I am feeling triggered by what was just said, I need a few minutes, can we please discuss this in twenty minutes? I am not walking away from you, what you have to say is important to me but I need a bit of time."

Partner 2:

> "Ok, that sounds like a plan. Let's come back and talk about it again when you are ready. What you have to say is important to me too and I would like to hear your thoughts."

So, in twenty minutes when both parties are ready to talk, you can do so in a more calm and less triggered state. You can discuss why you were triggered, how you felt when you were triggered and what you heard your partner say. Your partner can clarify what exactly they meant and validate your feelings. Miscommunication and the way in which our message has been perceived needs to be brought out into the open. Hopefully by being understood, the problem is resolved and irradicated. Remember that underneath that iceberg of triggered emotions, there is always an unmet need. If you can be vulnerable with your partner, communicate effectively to work through your trigger and how you are feeling, that need will become more clear, and therefore a lot easier to meet.

"Help comes to those who have the courage to ask for it."

Author unknown

Chapter 5

Asking For Help

In order to take the best care of your marriage you *must* take care of yourself. You can't be a useful participant in a strong partnership if you don't keep yourself in check and healthy. If you have high expectations of your partner, you should have high expectations of yourself as well. I am talking about your physical health and your mental health. If you are not taking care of yourself, how on earth do you expect to take care of something as precious as your marriage? You can't...*period!* And if you say you can, you, your marriage, or both will falter. How do I say this with such conviction? I see it in my clients when they first come in and I can also speak from first-hand experience. My first marriage was so out of balance and our priorities were so off kilter that they slowly eroded and a wrecking ball of destruction finished off what little we had left standing.

Health has always been a priority to me. Health is so important to your overall well-being, that it affects every aspect of your life. If you do not have your health, what do you have? I think of it as a precious gift that you give to yourself and to your family. If you pay attention to your health by listening to your body, and what it needs, it generally responds with gratitude. Sometimes we get derailed and things happen that throw us off the tracks but with help such as consistency, and in some cases medical professionals, we most often get can back on track and keep rolling.

When you are in a marriage or a relationship where health is not a priority for you or your other half, it can be challenging on the best of days. I was often belittled or was made to feel shameful for what I chose to eat or for the choices that I made to keep myself healthy. Often people project what they are battling onto the people who are closest to them. You know you the best, you know what your body needs and wants if you take the time to listen. When you fail to listen to the whispers, they become louder and louder. Eventually they scream in your face for your undivided attention and can deeply impact your entire life.

My message here is that everyone needs help at some point. No one, and I mean no one reaches their goal without some sort of help. It doesn't matter if your goal is to be the CEO of a large cooperation, if it is to learn how to play a new sport, or if it is to have a super successful marriage, we cannot get there without the help of many. If you take a solid look at your relationship right now, there will be a list of names of people who have offered support or given support in some fashion along the way. If your relationship is still pretty new, just know that year after year that list will grow. So, the act of asking for help from people who have already paved the path, or could make our path less bumpy should not be frowned upon. The rate of marriage breakdowns and divorce would be cut drastically if there wasn't such a stigma about asking or needing some guidance from professionals who are more than happy to help us reach our goals. Research shows that couples wait up to six years to seek help which could have been resolved in a much shorter time frame if they had just reached out sooner. According to The Gottman Institute (2020), only 19 percent of couples seek professional support and guidance. The longer we wait to ask for help the more desperate, isolated, and frustrated we become. When feelings are not worked through and solutions are not found, needs are not met. What happens when needs are not met? More conflict arises and when more conflict arises, the less connected and safe we feel as the downward spiral continues.

There is no shame in asking for or needing help. This lesson took me way too long to learn and it could have saved a lot of heartache and a lot of hard lessons. If you have questions that are unanswered or if you are frustrated after trying the same things over and over, *ask* for help. Even if you feel like you are drowning and need support, you need to listen to your inner voice and give it what it needs. The end result will get you to your goal a lot faster with a lot less trips and falls along the way.

I often compare it to buying a piece of furniture from IKEA. We've probably all done it or have heard stories about bringing the box home and putting the new masterpiece together. First of all, my dear friend D has always said that this is a great potential or future partner test and should be a premarital prerequisite, which I think is brilliant... but I digress. So, back to the furniture, in all its disassembled glory, unboxed and ready to be put together. What is the best way to tackle this project as a couple? Well, of course paying someone is a great option, if you wanted to but that isn't what I am getting at here. Reading the directions that came with your purchase would be the best solution here, right? Even with the instructions included, some projects are more difficult to put together with the fragments and bits that you are given. And don't you find that there are always extra pieces leftover that make you question your more than stellar construction skills? Depending on what season your marriage is going through, it can be a delightful walk in the park or it could feel like you want to rip your hair out, that too much elbow grease, frustration or anger are being exerted. Since we aren't handed a manual of instructions, like most projects, when we sign our marriage license, we need to keep our options open. If something comes up along the way that we are struggling with, the option is there to reach out and ask for guidance, support and some useful tools to add to the marriage/relationship/sex toolbox. As an intimacy coach and clinical sexologist, this is what I love to do, this is my mission.

When there is intentional work put in, and both sides of the partnership can get on the same page, some incredible changes can and will unfold. When you can optimize your relationship environment outside of the bedroom, it is a lot easier to make things happen inside of the bedroom. Amazing sex lives don't just happen, just like you don't fall into an amazing marriage. You *both* made it that way and if you want it to stay amazing then you have to put in the time and the work to get it there and keep it there. You don't just plant a garden and then reap the benefits for years to come by just gazing out the window at it every once in a blue moon. No! You have to have a plan and stick to it. You need to water it, you need to pick the weeds, you need to fertilize, tend to it, and put some love into the process. Then and only then will you see the fruits of your labor.

The same goes for your relationship and your sex life. When a few weeds pop up, you don't say, "Screw it, I'm done." No. You get out there, get your hands dirty and do what you need to do to get it to where it needs to be to flourish and thrive. All relationships go through difficult times and all sex lives do too. The storms that we sometimes feel when we are in a challenging spot in our relationship can only last for so long. The light eventually appears through the darkness and the more we focus on the light, the more light we see. The more weeds we pick, the more room we have to grow and shine together.

Do not second-guess yourself or feel ashamed or weak for needing help or extra guidance. Those who have the courage to ask for what they need are those who are given the tools to navigate their way to a more fulfilling relationship and sex life. Think about your life in general. You have always needed help and asked for guidance or an extra hand for many tasks. It could have been when you were working on a certain project for school or creating a proposal for a prospective client. We rarely do anything completely on our own.

We enlist the help of our family, of friends, of colleagues, of contractors, even of the good old internet. If everyday jobs and tasks are easy to enlist the help of others on and it is even expected in a lot of cases, why would you all of a sudden not need any help when it comes to your marriage? It doesn't make any sense. We are just supposed to figure it out on our own? That is crazy and it doesn't have to be this way. There are many of us out there who would love to help. That way, the tools and techniques to help make the speed bumps and the hurdles easier to conquer, are ready to be utilized whenever they are needed. There is no shame in asking for help. It is an act of courage and ensures that life will be a lot more smooth and enjoyable!

It's time to crack open your workbook. I want to give you the opportunity to brainstorm for just a few minutes. You and your spouse are asked to take just five or ten minutes to make a list of those who have supported you and your relationship along the way. It is rather enlightening to become aware of the vast number of people who have helped you, as a couple. People, even those who we don't think too much about, help you and your family every single day. Who helps to ensure your family has nourishing food on the table on a daily basis? Yes, of course, you do but who makes sure the shelves are stocked and that food actually gets to your grocery stores? Who helps to keep your family healthy? Here is a small sample of ideas to get your minds rolling.

Who has helped you?

- Friends
- Family
- Pastor/Reverend/Priest/Rabbi
- Sexologist
- Counselor
- Coach
- Bible Study Leader
- Teacher
- Plumber
- Real Estate Agent
- Electrician
- Home Builder
- Boss

- Colleague
- Nurse
- Grocery Store Clerk
- Farmers
- Truck Drivers
- Doctors
- Dentists
- Hairstylist
- Dog Walker
- Day Care Employee(s)
- Personal Trainer
- Authors
- Police Officer
- EMT/Firefighter
- Restaurant Employees
- Clothing Store Employees
- Pharmacist

The list could actually go on for pages and pages but hop into your workbook and have a chat about the people who have lent a helping hand in your direction. When we take the time to shine a light on those who have had an impact on you, it is quite remarkable.

"Intimacy – when you find it cherish it, take the utmost care of it because it is one of the most precious gifts that you will ever experience."

Shauna Harris

Chapter 6

Types of Intimacy

When we think of the word intimacy, the vast majority of people associate it with sex. While this is not inaccurate in any sense of the word, it is just a small part of the definition. Sex is for sure a part of the intimacy puzzle but there are a number of other pieces that need to fit into the equation as well.

Intimacy comes in many forms, so if we can begin by understanding each piece of this puzzle, we can more easily create a balance in our lives. Our marriage or relationship will be set up for the forever scenario. When we look at intimacy as a whole picture, it can tend to be daunting. Stories may begin to play in our minds and we might tell ourselves, "It has been too long since we were on the same page to get back to a happy place" or, "I don't even know where to start." Well, sometimes when we bite off a little chunk at a time instead of inhaling the entire meal, it is much easier to digest. Let me clarify it for you and show you what I am talking about.

Intimacy can be broken down into bite-sized pieces as follows:

1. Intellectual intimacy
2. Recreational intimacy
3. Financial intimacy

4. Spiritual intimacy
5. Emotional intimacy
6. Physical intimacy

If we can look at each of these bites individually, it helps to explain the complexity of all that encompasses intimacy. Once we can better understand the different forms, increasing the level of intimacy in our relationships doesn't seem so staggering a goal to reach. One step at a time is the name of the game!

Intellectual intimacy is coming together, freely sharing our thoughts and ideas with our partner. We don't always share the same opinion. Having intellectual intimacy allows us to be comfortable to express our differences in the areas that are important in our relationship. Being able to talk to our partner about virtually anything and respecting each other's views and opinions help to build a foundation of trust and support. Whether it be health, cooking, future goals, philosophy, literature, etc, our interests, thoughts and knowledge can spark the deepest of conversations and can bring the two of you into a more intimate place.

Recreational intimacy can be described simply as the time spent doing activities and going to various places together. It also includes the everyday tasks and time spent together as well. Spending time with one another is so important in increasing the level of intimacy in relationships. The time spent together creates memories, adds excitement, and also incorporates the element of fun. We all know how we feel when we are having fun. It feels really good! This could mean doing activities that both of you love. It could be exploring new activities, or enjoying an activity that is new to one of you and encourages the other to try. Any event that has the two of you spending time together fits under recreational intimacy. It could be traveling, volunteering, going to a concert or a festival, exercising, taking the dog for a walk, wine tasting, even video games.

When was the last time you had fun together? It doesn't really matter what you do as a couple, just make sure it is enjoyable and maybe switch it up once and awhile! I have so many date ideas, 110 to be exact, listed in the next chapter for you to consider if you are in need of some ideas or just need a little boost to spark your creativity. Check them out and see what you might want to add to your "Date Ideas List" to try in the very near future. They range from super simple to some that are a little over the top, so that everyone could find a few nuggets that they might be interested in and might be willing to try. You could even step out of your comfort zone and attempt something wild and crazy. The dopamine, serotonin and oxytocin will start rushing through your body when you try something new together and then look out! Those happy hormones are known to flip that intimacy switch and start to build those positive emotions, resulting in you feeling more connected with one another.

Financial intimacy seems to muster up some pain points and tends to push some uncomfortable buttons for some. This is completely normal and is a great opportunity, as a team, to work through and conquer those uncomfortable spots together. When you are looking to increase the financial intimacy in your marriage you are working toward being comfortable in the sharing of your finances and your financial situation. Financial intimacy can mean discussing a budget but it is much more than this. It is discussing your financial goals and a financial plan; it is having a healthy relationship with money and your partner. There needs to be a level of mutual respect, shared control, equality, and a common vision. One spouse may have a higher income but you are both on the same team. Financial decisions should and need to be made together.

We come into any relationship or marriage with different views on money so we need to spend the time to learn to work together. It is important to talk about each other's spending habits and to come up with a plan that works for both of you. How does a joint account benefit your marriage and should you have separate accounts as well? What about credit cards? How many and what will they be used for? Is there a plan for paying them off every month? Who will be the designated bill payer? Will you do it together? Should you split the tasks? Maybe one of you has a love for numbers or accounting. This is where your strength may come in handy. Use your strengths! Financial intimacy is a critical part of your overall intimacy, as it develops trust. Trust develops feelings of being supported, of feeling safe, and of truly being on the same page as our partner. When you can tackle challenges by working together to become a united front it is a powerful bonding experience that really can strengthen your relationship.

Spiritual intimacy is all about sharing beliefs and religious practices and valuing the differences that each of you share. Mutual respect and trust are essential to increase and maintain spiritual intimacy. We all grew up in very different homes with very different parents/guardians, different family dynamics, different practices, and very different traditions. No two people come into any type of relationship having the exact same belief system or religious customs. Being accepting of who each of you is on your spiritual journey is absolutely necessary. Having an open mind to discuss where each partner is on their individual journey and where they want to go will help keep conflict at bay.

Ask yourselves, "How are we spiritual together?" Many of us have a clear direction of where we are going and what path we are choosing to take while others might not have a clue about what spirituality even means to them. As a couple, it is a powerful piece to the entire intimacy puzzle. If you can find a common ground or a common understanding of where you both want to go together, this will bind you and connect you even further. Some ideas to try with your partner or continue to do as a couple are: pray together, attend church together, sign up for a couples' Bible study, practice yoga, meditate together, read a spiritual book together or listen to podcasts together. This is just a small list of ideas to increase your spiritual intimacy but these might just inspire you to start the conversation of developing a plan of action for the two of you.

I have very deliberately left over the last two types of intimacy as the final two pieces to discuss. Why, you may ask? Well, all six of these intimacy pieces are extremely interconnected but these two seem to generate the most clients and questions in my practice. Please remember: they are all incredibly important to embrace and to incorporate in your relationship, if you are seeking a seriously solid foundation to sail into that unchartered and untraveled voyage of forever.

Emotional intimacy happens when a relationship feels safe and secure enough to be open and vulnerable. The word vulnerable can evoke some pretty strong emotions, even from the most chill and relaxed individual. People tend to come from two different camps when it comes to this word. You are either on team, "Hell, yes!" or team "Hell no, but thanks for asking!" The people who are "open books" and who have no problem answering when asked personal questions, obviously have few hurdles building up this type of intimacy. The distance of the road between these two camps differs for each individual — some can be persuaded down the path with the right words and the right environment. There must be a feeling of safety and acceptance, with no judgment. Just because you reside in or are very comfortable in one camp, doesn't mean that you can't switch attitudes, even for those people who have a solid padlock on their vulnerability door.

There are many different reasons emotional intimacy is difficult for some people. We are all a product of our experiences and when there has been trauma or negative events, it is easier to seal that part of ourselves to keep us safe and unexposed. When we allow oursel to slowly show our vulnerability in an environment that we create with our partner that is comfortable, inviting, and non-threatening, it is such a great sense of freedom that feels like a million pounds being lifted off of our frame. The walls that we have built to keep us "safe" can come crumbling down when there is a sense of security and support for one another's strengths and weaknesses. Sharing each other's aspirations, needs, desires, thoughts, and feelings creates a bond and increases the level of emotional intimacy in the relationship. Emotional intimacy creates an atmosphere of trust. To maintain it, both partners need to ensure that they are emotionally available and willing to find the time to have meaningful conversations and to value what each other has to offer. When you can count on your spouse to be there, to be accessible when you need them and when they need you, magic happens with your level of emotional intimacy.

Last but definitely not least, is our level of **physical intimacy**. When I ask couples about certain aspects of their physical intimacy, more often than not they default to sex and their sex lives. Yes, physical intimacy has everything to do with your sex life but it is not just about sex. It encompasses a whole lot more. It is the touching and the close proximity to one another. This includes holding hands, hugging, kissing, caressing, cuddling, massaging, any kind of touching as well as sexual activity. As humans, we thrive on physical contact. It has even been proven to increase the strength of our immune system. I do agree that some individuals are more "touchy" than others, so the amount of touching will vary from couple to couple and it all comes down to what works for you and your partner. I so highly recommend that you make it a point to touch each other non-sexually every single day. This is particularly important if you are looking to increase the level of satisfaction in your sex life.

Our largest organ in the body is our skin and when it is touched, our nervous system is activated and sends various signals to our brain. Our brain then releases oxytocin, dopamine, and serotonin, which as I mentioned before are our feel good hormones. These hormones make us feel really great and in turn, we also feel an increased sense of connection with our partner. While these happy hormones are being released, our brain sends a message to our stress hormones to diminish or to stop being released. Yup, these stress hormones, such as cortisol and norepinephrine, get the "back off" message which is such a welcomed gift for your body. Cortisol is our "fight-or-flight" hormone.

It is responsible for increasing our heart rate and our blood pressure when we are feeling stressed out. We all know and feel what happens in our bodies when we are stressed. There is definitely a time and a place for cortisol and it is essential in our bodies but when it is released in excess over a period of time, it can cause weight gain, accelerated aging, it messes with our sleep patterns, it decreases the effectiveness of our immune system and that is just to name a few. So, when I say that it is the little things every day that can make the biggest difference, this is one of those little things. It is a really great habit to get into when you intentionally reach out and grab your hubby's butt or give him a little smooch as you walk by or give your wife a little snuggle or rub her back. It doesn't take a huge amount of effort but the payoffs inside and out are more than meets the eye.

Being willing to talk about the level of physical intimacy in your relationship is a good sign that you and your partner will get on the same page and stay there. When you are able to talk about sex, your sex life will be more satisfying. Those who routinely talk about sex, (and I highly suggest it, in fact) have better sex lives. I want to give you some peace of mind here. You are not alone if sex is a difficult topic to bring up or talk about with your partner. Most people find it uncomfortable and awkward. Some have never brought it up at all and they have been together for a really long time. It is no wonder that a lot of people struggle in this area, as so many of us were given such negative messages about sex growing up. It doesn't help that the sex education in North America is so basic and that it gets more bare bones every year.

When I used to teach Human Sexuality, over twenty years ago, it was a lot more extensive than it is now and that isn't saying much. We are expected to make informed decisions about sex and our sexual health but if we aren't informed the way we should be and need to be, how can we make the most educated decisions? *We can't.* A big part of my practice is educating teens. In today's world, much of the information on sexual behavior is gained secondhand through apps, movies, text messaging, and friends. Exaggeration, misinformation, or limited knowledge about sex and relationships is confusing and sometimes hard to differentiate between fact and fiction. Factual information is essential to help set our kids up for a positive and healthy sex life. If young adults venture into the world with a solid foundation and knowledge-base, they are more likely to make well-informed, educated decisions. Sex can be an awkward and uncomfortable topic to discuss; we struggle to find the words with our partners, let alone our kids.

Talking about sex does involve some risk on our part at first, because we don't want to be judged, or criticized. We may feel insecure or silly, and we definitely don't want to be rejected. We often associate sex with shame or shameful feelings and we need to reframe that thought process. Sex was designed for us to enjoy and to enjoy each other. If sex is difficult for you to talk about with your partner, start with simple questions that make you curious. Talking about sex is also easier when you are not engaged in the act. Going for a walk or a drive makes couples less self-conscious when there is some sort of neutral activity involved. I have some great tips and techniques in this department that makes talking about sex less awkward, more fun, and a whole lot more enjoyable. Because sex is such an intimate act, it can be extremely difficult to talk about. We tend to overthink the situation and let our insecurities creep in. Those insecurities end up pitching a tent and staying awhile. No one needs that and if we view our partner as our best friend, we need to work towards treating them as such. We need to give them the benefit of the doubt that they will have our backs and want to work together towards a mind-blowing sex life.

We all have ideas or thoughts that we allow to fester and grow and we shouldn't. It could be a fear of being rejected, or performance anxiety, or we may think that we look undesirable or maybe those extra pounds are at the forefront of our minds. We might even be thinking that we should have shaved or had a shower before jumping in the sack. Whatever comes up for you, just allow your mind to go to a place where, if you had the ideal situation to just talk about it, you would. Those insecurities or worries that creep in and take over would soon melt away because your partner would have nothing but support, love, and encouragement for you. This is where you are headed because when you make it a point to put your sex life on the ongoing topic list, nothing is off the table. It can be so freeing to bring up a desire that you have dreamed about or, if something wasn't quite working for you mid-session, it becomes no big deal to change things up with a quick lil' comment or an adjustment on your part.

Sex, when freely talked about, can't help but get better. Again, I am a testament to this tried and tested equation. In my first marriage I had no idea why sex was not discussed. When I look back, it even seems silly to me now how much it was avoided. I wasn't interested in talking about sex. I was insecure about my body when I had nothing to be insecure about. We never asked each other what we wanted, what we liked, what we needed, what we desired. I can remember talking about sexual fantasies a few times but that was easy for me because they seemed somehow not in the realm of reality and I could separate myself from the awkwardness of the conversation. It is sad really, but on the flip side, I wouldn't be helping to educate individuals and couples reach their sexuality goals if I hadn't gone through and learned all that I have learned.

When you go from one sexual environment to another that is so polar opposite, as I have, it is extremely eye-opening for one, but holy dynamite, it is refreshing. It makes it crystal clear how extremely important communication is in a relationship and how deeply it affects life between the sheets. I wasted so much time keeping my mouth shut and trying to avoid confrontation or whatever I was protecting myself from at the time. When you have a willing partner who is so open to discuss absolutely anything, it is hard not to rock it in the sex life department. When one is made to feel completely safe, protected, taken care of, supported, loved, and confident, conversation and trust flows so much easier. When a topic isn't made to be a big deal to talk about, it just isn't. We need to work together as couples to be all of this and more. Watch what happens to your sexual desire and your sex life.

Anything worth having needs regular maintenance, time, care and attention, just like the garden that I discussed before. It doesn't matter if it's a garden, a car, a home, a bank account, a friend, or a partner; if we don't nurture it, it will not thrive. I often equate it with the legs of a stool or a chair. If one is not balanced with the others or maintained, the entire stability of the structure is off. Taking the time to work on the six kinds of intimacy will propel your relationship far into the future. Making the effort to maintain and care for the intimacy levels in your relationship will not only become habitual but it will be so rewarding and your sex life will thank you for it.

"A great marriage is not when the 'perfect couple' comes together. It is when an imperfect couple learns to enjoy their differences."

Dave Meuer

Chapter 7

Date Night

One of the most effective tools in your "Couple's Tool-box" needs to be *Date Night!* This crazy lil' tool works in magical ways that you may not have even thought of. A special designated time, set aside once a week or once every two weeks, is a crucial piece of the intricate puzzle that couples create piece by piece as they build their relationship together.

Incorporating this gem does wonders to the level of intimacy that we all need and crave in our lives. Making an effort and a commitment to spend quality time engaging in conversation while enjoying each other over a meal, going for a walk, or a hike, brings couples closer and re-establishes their bond.

It doesn't really matter what you choose to do. It's the "doing" of the date that counts. If coming up with ideas makes you cringe or makes your brain hurt, no worries, I can help you out in that area. I have included a list of ideas below that you can use as a springboard to create other ideas. Make sure you switch things up though. Going to the same restaurant each week, picking the same meal and enjoying the same dessert might sound delicious and you might even be salivating but after a while, it also sounds dull and safe. We weren't born to be dull people, so get out there and shine. Going new places and doing new things together increases dopamine (the happy hormone) and that's a really good thing. When you are experiencing new things with your guy or girl it is a new level of shaking things up or adding some spice.

In your *Speaking of Sex Workbook,* I have included a list for each of you. I would love for you both to highlight the ideas that pique your interest and those that are your favorites. It is really interesting and often turns into a great discussion when each partner does this activity on their own. When you are both finished highlighting the dates that sound like your idea of a good time, come back and compare your lists. Talk about why you chose the dates that you did and why you would find them enjoyable. Most couples learn something new about their partners and it can be exhilarating to have a few fun activities to look forward to. Some of these ideas you may not be able to do at the moment. I completely understand this but I would like you to have a few new ideas to begin to plan for in the future. It is a great little exercise to do together. Your *Date Night* list is included below but remember to check out your workbook to complete the activity.

Which of the ideas below would you like to try one day soon? Let the adventurous part of your mind take you for a ride!

1. Go for a long walk.
2. Work out together.
3. Make a meal together.
4. Check out a new restaurant.
5. Go for a hike.
6. Catch a movie.
7. Go to a comedy show.

8. Take a Bible Study or a spiritual class.
9. See a play.
10. Take a dance class.
11. Go away for a weekend.
12. Explore a local tourist attraction.
13. Go bowling.
14. Try mini golfing.
15. Check out your local farmer's market.
16. Attend a book reading.
17. Set up a mini scavenger hunt for your partner.
18. Take your honey to a football game.
19. Christmas shop together.
20. Tour model homes in your area.
21. Go grocery shopping together.
22. Try batting cages.
23. Go on a picnic.
24. Get tickets for a basketball game.
25. Horseback ride.
26. Take a wine tasting tour.
27. Get some of your favorite ice cream together.
28. Swim.
29. Go see a baseball game.
30. Take a cooking class together.
31. Practice yoga.
32. Get a couple's massage.
33. Go to a concert.
34. Volunteer at a local food kitchen.
35. Take in a hockey game.
36. Drive to a nearby town and act like tourists.
37. Go for coffee or tea.

38. Find a little bakery for a yummy treat.
39. Go to the museum.
40. Star gaze in your back yard or at a nearby park.
41. Test drive your dream car.
42. Go camping.
43. Board or card game night.
44. Rent canoes or a boat.
45. Take in a Karaoke night.
46. Try a self-defense class.
47. Go for a bike ride.
48. Build a snowman.
49. Go sledding.
50. Have a candlelight bath.
51. Plant a small herb garden.
52. Re-create your first date.
53. Go listen to live music.
54. Do a food truck tour.
55. Go to the spa.
56. Take a pottery class.
57. Go ice skating.
58. Head for the carnival.
59. Find a cool dive bar.
60. Hit the driving range.
61. Create a "bucket list" together.
62. Attend a charity event.
63. Visit a local animal shelter and snuggle with the dogs.
64. Go to a nearby farm and pick some fruit/veggies.
65. Volunteer together.
66. Take a hot air balloon ride.

67. Visit a local State Park and explore.
68. Spar with a few boxing lessons.
69. Visit the aquarium.
70. Go to the casino.
71. Take a helicopter tour of your city.
72. Carve a Halloween pumpkin.
73. Toast the pumpkin seeds.
74. Try out each other's favorite hobby.
75. Go to an escape room.
76. Try paintball.
77. Check out your local flea market.
78. Bake your favorite cookies or treat together.
79. Go to the zoo.
80. Check out an art show.
81. Go to a drive-in movie.
82. Make breakfast in bed.
83. Go to the waterpark.
84. Wash the cars on the driveway and get drenched.
85. Plant a tree in your yard and watch it grow together.
86. Explore a sex toy shop.
87. Have a snowball fight.
88. Play a game of laser tag.
89. Go lingerie shopping.
90. Visit an international or specialty grocery store.
91. Find each other a book to read in your local bookstore.
92. Play a few games of tennis.
93. Go to a food festival.
94. Head to the lake.

95. Get tattoos.
96. Go go-carting.
97. Visit an arcade and play some old school games.
98. Make a DYI project.
99. Hire a photographer to take some fun pics of you together.
100. Play Frisbee in the park.
101. Have a BBQ.
102. Go scuba diving.
103. Go fishing.
104. Play some pool at your local pub.
105. Make homemade ice cream.
106. Learn a new skill together (piano, guitar, etc.)
107. Check out your local fish or meat market.
108. Decorate the house for the holidays.
109. Write a romantic letter to each other and read it out loud to one another.
110. Spend a night in a hotel.

A little side note for you:

If you have kiddos, don't use them as an excuse to get out of *Date Night* either. We all have been guilty of making excuses or letting "life" get in the way. The weeks and months just start to fly by without notice. *Nope!* Not happening. Don't let that happen.

Instead:

1. Enlist the help of family to come and watch your little muffins.
2. Exchange babysitting duties with trusted friends. One week you watch their kiddos and then the next week they watch yours. This could

turn out to be a fun night with your spouse too, make it fun.

3. Maybe you already have a regular babysitter and this is a non-issue for *Date Night!* Lucky you!

4. Ask around the community to see if anyone knows a reliable sitter who could help you out on a regular basis.

5. Or…best case scenario, use a combo of the suggestions above to get out there and make some memories with your love!

If you can incorporate *Date Night* into your regular routine, if you can commit to this one-on-one time with your partner; it will be one of the best investments that you will ever make. It will also be one of the greatest gifts that you can *ever* give to your kiddos. Having parents who have fun together and enjoy each other's company is a gift that keeps giving. You are building a firm foundation on which your relationship will grow, flourish, and last well into your golden years.

"The basic conflict between men and women sexually, is that men are like fireman. To men, sex is an emergency and no matter what we're doing we can be ready in two minutes. Women, on the other hand, are like fire. They're very exciting but the conditions have to be exactly right for it to occur."

Jerry Seinfeld

Chapter 8

Sexual Satisfaction

Now that we are well-versed in the different types of intimacy, and some ways in which we can work as a team with our partner to increase and maintain the level of intimacy in all six areas, I want to take things a step further. It's time to talk about how you can work together, as a couple, and how you can begin to have a massive impact in the level of satisfaction in your sex life. I know I just got your attention didn't I? This actually is where the fun part of the "work" comes in!

We all know that men and women respond differently when turned on or when they are interested in having sex. Our bodies are created very differently and therefore are going to respond very differently. So many of my clients come to me to address this very thing, as it is a very common concern or issue that many couples have. One spouse typically has a higher desire than the other. It is a common misconception that the male is always the higher desire and the woman is the lower desire. This is not always the case. It is even very normal for partners to alternate every now and then. What I want to do here is help you understand the differences between the male and the female sexual response cycles.

Why We Are So Different

There are so many variables that can and do affect your libido. It can be something as simple as fatigue but it can also be affected by more serious situations, such as a medical condition. Our sexual desires are susceptible to change on a dime and our health definitely plays a big part in keeping our sexual health at an optimal state and at a level in which you are content with. Here is just a small list of things that will have an impact on your desire to have sex:

- high blood pressure
- coronary artery disease
- diabetes
- certain prescription drugs
- neurological diseases
- birth control
- stress
- sleep patterns
- exercise
- nutrition
- personality
- hormone levels
- level of intimacy in your relationship
- alcohol intake
- illicit drug use
- unresolved conflict
- low level of trust with your partner
- poor communication

- performance anxiety
- body image issues
- past trauma
- erectile dysfunction
- vaginal dryness
- painful past sexual experience
- difficulty orgasming

If you and your spouse can make some healthy adjustments to your day-to-day lives, it will have a positive impact on your libido. If there is a medical issue, the best route to take here is to seek the guidance and advice from your doctor. When you come to the table with a clean bill of health, or at least an understanding of how your condition(s) is making an impact on your sex life, you can move into the educational part of the equation to help better understand yourself and your spouse.

I am going to first talk about and describe what happens in the male body and then I will explain what happens in the female body. The purpose here is for us to understand that we were not created the same way and therefore we cannot expect the other person to respond the same or even in a similar way. I also want to make sure that you know that there are exceptions to every rule but this does and will ring true to the majority. These two charts below have been adapted from LMFT, Sam Tielemans (2020).

All right men, let's get to it. When we take a look at the sexual response that occurs within the bodies of the men in our lives, it is a pretty simple and easy to understand the linear sequence of events. There is usually some sort of stimulus that sets this process in motion. Males are typically very visual beings, so more than likely they have seen something that they are fond of and this leads them to the desire stage. The desire stage then moves to a state of arousal, and then orgasm usually results.

Of course, this can be stated in a more clinical and scientific manner but I want to keep things straightforward. My goal is for us to understand how each other's bodies function so that we are more aware going forward. When we are more aware, we are more willing to show up with compassion and support one another. The more we understand each other on every level, the easier the degree of intimacy can elevate because there is less room for miscommunication and misunderstanding.

Another bit of information that needs to be mentioned here is that after an orgasm has occurred, there is a refractory period. This is the phase in which the body needs to recover. The length of time that the body needs to relax and recover after climax differs in everyone but it is referred to as the resting state where muscles relax, heart rate and blood pressure return to their normal state and the body is less responsive to any further sexual stimulation. In the male body however, it is a typically longer refractory period than in the female body. Many sources suggest that women don't even have a refractory period. On the other hand, most claim that women indeed do report a brief period of time in which their body needs a second or two before they can continue with sexual activity. Men can take anywhere from a few minutes to a day or two before the body is able to be aroused again and this is affected by a variety of factors that include diet, exercise habits, libido, and overall health. The little diagram that I have included on the next page shows just how linear the male response is.

Male Response

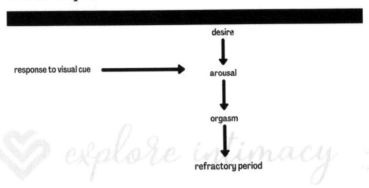

I want to mention here that I have included orgasm in this picture but please note that an orgasm doesn't always occur and doesn't have to occur with every sexual experience to make it great. We can feel fulfilled, loved, and satisfied without reaching climax every time. Society likes to make us believe that unless we are swinging from the chandelier and generating decibel-shattering screams of our partner's name during an orgasm, that the sexual encounter wasn't up to par. This needs to be wiped out and permanently deleted from our minds. We need to write our own definition of satisfying sex. Does it feel good? Is it fun? Are we connecting in a meaningful way with our significant other? Men and women both have been led to believe that unless they orgasm and help to make their partner orgasm, they are not preforming between the sheets. It takes a lot more than a straight line to make a woman climax so my hope in educating you on the differences between males and females in this area, is that as a couple you can both create an environment where an orgasm is possible and attainable whenever you want it to be.

Ok ladies, you're up! Women tend to be a bit more complex in the sexual response cycle. There are a few more steps involved before she is even at a point of desiring sexual intimacy. Women tend to start in a very neutral space when it comes to wanting sex and in order for them to want to proceed to the next step of desire, a few stars need to be aligned. This is where men can come into play and can encourage their wives and even speed up this process. There could even be a hard "no" on her lips but with a few intentional actions and/ or words exchanged between a couple, it can flip the switch and she can decide to engage in sex, if she feels so inclined. What our male counterparts might not realize is that so much of what it takes for women to jump in full throttle is what is happening between her ears, not between her thighs.

Let's start with the current state of the relationship. How has the climate been recently? If it is in a good place, you are one step closer to the bedroom for sure. Simply stated, without an emotional connection, there is a lack of sexual desire in women. It is easier for women to feel "turned on" or to be "turned on" when they feel safe and secure in their relationship. If they are feeling connected and safe in their relationship, it is a lot easier for them to move to the next step in the sexual response cycle.

The frontal cortex (the very front section) of a woman's brain is very much involved in the decision for her to want sex. She must actually make the decision that she is going to have sex for things to proceed to desire. It all starts with a decision! Women pair together safety concerns with sexual response. They subconsciously make a decision to have sex based on the reasoning and control center of their brain. Men, when they do not understand this or are not made aware of this, get frustrated. This is understandable because they don't need to subconsciously have all of these things in order to have an increase in desire and have sex. When men are turned on, it's go time!

When a woman feels that sense of safety and connection with her partner, there is a release of oxytocin in her body. When oxytocin is present, it shuts off her "fight-or-flight" response and promotes feelings of trust. We want and have the desire to connect and be closer to our spouse. When trust is generated, safety and closeness is felt and sex is more likely to happen. When sex occurs, even more oxytocin is released and the cycle continues. So when a husband or partner has ever been frustrated with their wife or partner and has uttered, "You never want to have sex," or something along those lines, a different way of thinking or a changed perspective may be in order. How about asking yourself, "What is the state of our relationship right now and how can I make her feel more connected and safe with me right now?" Amazing things can happen when we first take the time to connect. We need to start by creating an environment of trust so that women can feel this sense of safety and want to connect on a deeper level with their partner.

Now let's take a look at the Female Response Cycle. As mentioned, there are a few more steps in this cycle compared to the male cycle that we just looked at above. The climate of the relationship, the level of safety and connections or emotional intimacy matters to a female. Even a recent sexual experience that may not have gone as planned or left her with some unfulfilled needs, unexpressed needs, or certain emotions may be affecting her present state. It might take a conversation to make her feel more connected and supported. Once she feels connected to her partner, she is then in the clear to feel the desire for sex. When a woman finds herself approaching this stage, her state of arousal is highly dependent on sexual cues from her partner. This isn't to say she can't, shouldn't, and doesn't take the lead here or doesn't initiate because that is also important. What I am saying is that in order for her to move from desire to arousal, she is taking cues from her partner and the way in which he responds.

A lot of males like to "go for the goods" right away and this is another difference between most males and females. Because a lady takes a little bit of time to warm up (and this certainly varies for each individual), she will respond more quickly if she is given some time to be aroused. This is often referred to as foreplay and the amount of time that she needs here is not a particular number of minutes. It fluctuates from day to day and is ever-changing. Some women take just a couple of minutes and some can take over 20 minutes to get to where they need to be, depending on the day, the state of the relationship, how she is feeling, etc. Men are like microwaves and women are like ovens. They need to preheat before they are ready to go, so take the time and have some fun with foreplay. Foreplay doesn't have to start in the bedroom. It can start the minute you wake up in the morning and last the entire day, if that is what tickles your fancy. Be creative, have fun with it, switch it up and by the time you jump in between the sheets the state of arousal might be through the roof.

For comparison, here is the Female Response Cycle for you to take a look at and see the differences between the two:

Female Response

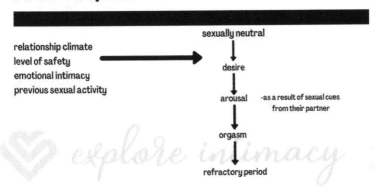

I know that I don't need to mention again about the fact that I included orgasm in the model but just to remind you, it doesn't necessarily need to be in there to have incredible sex with your partner. We do need to talk a bit more about the refractory period in women here though. A woman doesn't always need a long period of time to recover from climax. In a lot of sexual response diagrams, it is not even mentioned in the female cycle but it does vary from woman to woman. She may just need to a second to breathe and then she might be ready to go again and again.

Just to reiterate, the time will vary from woman to woman but she does have the incredible capability for multiple orgasms, if you both are up for the task. It can be a ton of fun exploring this little challenge. There are a lot of women who believe that they are not able to have one orgasm, let alone have multiple orgasms. I disagree. Women have the potential, when they can just be in the moment and enjoy themselves and their partner, to experience many different types of orgasms. You have to be a willing partner and have an open mind though. You may just surprise yourself! You wouldn't be the first to change your mind on this and you will definitely not be the last. The practical research is rather enjoyable. I highly recommend it.

Since we are on the subject of the "Big O," I want to discuss the prevalence of this in women in general. Most healthy men are not strangers to hittin' the big O, whether they are pleasuring themselves or are with their partner but a large percentage of women often find the goal of orgasm elusive and unattainable. Compared to men, women are considerably less likely to orgasm during heterosexual penetrative sex. In fact, reports find that up to 95 percent of men orgasm during sexual activity and women report a much lower rate, between 50 to 60 percent. If we could point fingers as to the reasons why there is such a vast difference between men and women, those fingers usually need to be pointing in the direction of what's going on in a woman's mind and what is currently going on in her relationship. Here we can go back to the importance of connection and feeling safe about where things are currently at between partners. The more connected and on the same page you are with your partner, the higher the chance of orgasm.

The mind plays a massive role in reaching orgasms and it isn't always working in her favor. Just as the frontal cortex plays a part in sexual desire, it is not the head cheerleader in the game of climaxing either. Rational thought decreases the ability to orgasm and being able to focus and train the female brain to let go of the cares of the day, to be in the moment, and try to shut out the world is such a great tool in getting closer to climax. A woman's self-esteem and how she feels about herself and her body play a role too, as does how well she and her partner communicate about sex in and out of the bedroom. Religious beliefs, past experiences, trauma, stress, and fatigue are factors here too and cannot be forgotten. Sleep is so important to overall health as is finding ways to relieve stress. If I were to pick and choose the most important elements here that increase the chances of women having an orgasm, it would be the climate and the level of communication and intimacy in your relationship. If your partner is feeling safe and confident where things are at, the more likely and the more quickly she is going to get out of her rational thoughts and enjoy what's happening in the moment to just let go.

Another point that I feel that I need to make is about the clitoris. Education can definitely be your best friend here for both men and women, if you are looking for more knowledge on how to feel pleasure or how to give pleasure. Many of us grew up believing that the clitoris consisted of the teeny button-like erogenous zone that was tucked nicely under the clitoral hood. It is located slightly above the opening of the urethra and the vagina. While this remains to be an accurate statement, this is just the very tip or head (the glans clitoris) of the structure and it actually extends deep into the woman's body and can be felt in different places of the vagina when it is penetrated. I have included a picture of a 3D model of the actual size of what women are working with. The head of the clitoris alone contains approximately 8 000 nerve endings (double that of the penis) and is the *only* body part in either the male or the female body that has the sole purpose and responsibility of giving pleasure.

This is what we need to understand about the clitoris: it generally likes to be stimulated gently and generally needs to be given some love to reach orgasm. Only about 6 percent of women always orgasm during penetrative sex. The number of women who need direct clitoral stimulation to reach orgasm is around 70 percent. Sexual preferences are extremely diverse when it comes to the clitoris, what she likes and dislikes, but it is clear that it is a very important part of the equation for a lot of women.

Here is the actual model of the clitoris that I use to show my clients. Although my hands are not large, you can see in the picture that the size of the clitoris is much bigger than most people with and without vulvas realize. The head of the clitoris, is pictured just below my index finger and then the clitoris continues up and back towards the rectum. The shaft of the clitoris (where my index finger is holding it on the top) is the area that can no longer be seen, as the rest of it resides inside of the female body. This structure can also be compared to an iceberg; there is so much more than what we can see and a lot of the magic is happening well beneath the surface. The shaft of the clitoris splits in half to form the paired crura and the vestibular bulbs. The vestibular bulbs are the two roundish shaped extensions and they actually sit on either side and extend through the vaginal canal and towards the anus. For those of you who are interested in knowing where the G-spot is located, it is believed to be the point where the vestibular bulbs meet and touch the anterior wall of the vagina. The actual size of the clitoris can vary in size, depending on the body, but the average size is said to be approximately 4 inches long.

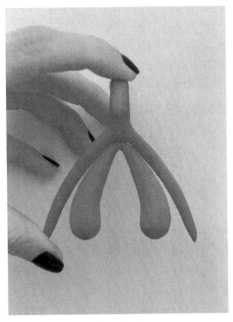

An interesting fact to know too is that as women age, the rate of orgasm actually increases. This is probably attributed to the fact that they are more comfortable with their bodies. Women become more in tune with their bodies, what they like as the years go by and are more willing to ask for what they want.

So now that we are aware of biological differences between a man and women in the sex response department, I want to explore further with you the differences that occur in the thought process between men and women sexually. We are all aware, for the most part, that we are wired differently but what we are not always aware of is that the way we are wired has an effect on the way we interact sexually. As we age, our thoughts evolve and the definition of satisfying sex evolves as well. When we become tuned in and can understand how our partner functions sexually and where they are coming from, it is a lot easier to be on the same page and work together. I need to mention that there are exceptions to each thought or statement made below. Our culture has pretty gender-specific beliefs on which pertain to males and which pertain to females but most of them are interchangeable.

Let's take the notion that there is always a high desire and a low desire person in every couple. It is believed that it is always the male who is the high desire when in fact stats show that this role changes throughout the relationship. When a woman feels sexually desirable, when she feels connected to her partner, comfortable and free to talk about sex, her desire increases. When women give themselves permission to be sexual beings, of which we all are, she is able to be more free and her desire for sex increases.

When it comes to being turned on visually, this typically goes to the male in the partnership. Men are extremely visual creatures but do not be mistaken, women are as well. The area of our brains, called the amygdala, which controls emotion and motivation, exhibits much higher levels of activation in the male brain when visual cues are present compared to the female brain. Scientists have summed this up to mean that the male then has to be the more visual of the two genders. I'd like to put a bit of a wrench in this theory because it is not that simple. Yes, men are highly sexually stimulated by visual cues and this is further illustrated in the Male Sexual Response Cycle that we talked about earlier in this chapter. My point here is that men process sexual visual cues very differently than females. Women's brain activity increases with visual cues as well but we have to take into account all of the other things that are happening at the same time. The Female Sexual Response Cycle also takes into account other factors that are occurring in her mind and in her body. What is the state of her hormones? What is her current status in the Response Cycle? If she is starting at neutral, she has a few steps to go before she is at the state of desire. She needs to make a decision that she is going to be sexual, whereas the men are more easily ready and raring to go.

Comparing men and women and their response to visual sexual stimuli is like comparing apples to oranges, that is they are both fruit, yes but made totally different. So, the old belief that women respond more mentally may very well be true but depending on what is going on in the male's world, he can and will respond in a more cognitive manner as well.

This leads us nicely into the next belief that women are more emotional and men are more physical. This one is pretty accurate but it does change as the relationship grows and matures. A women's desire is primarily emotional for sure and it is based on her emotional connection to her partner but it too can be more physical, just like men. It all depends on the individual and their current circumstances. The male's sexual desire, being primarily physical, does tend to evolve and become more emotional as time goes on so it doesn't remain a constant at all in any relationship. Because male sexual desire is more physical and for the majority of males, they are ready and raring to go at a moment's notice, a lot of men are known (as previously mentioned) to go, for lack of better words, "straight for the goods." When we are all aware of and understand the differences between the sexual response cycles, it helps our partners understand that women need a little revving of the engine. Women appreciate and sometimes need foreplay. They need their partner to take an indirect route to the "goods." Moving from sexually neutral to desire to arousal needs some persuading and sweet talking. Depending on the day, it could take a few seconds to 20 minutes as already mentioned. This alone could make a huge difference in your sex life. Foreplay can be and should be fun and rewarding. When done in a way that is pleasurable to you as a couple, this tool in your sexuality tool box can be a game changer.

Turn-ons/Turn-offs

Here is another example of where communication is so important. Wouldn't it be a lot easier to know exactly what each of you needed in the moment? It's a lot more fun when you aren't guessing what your partner likes and dislikes. Knowing each other's "turn-ons" and "turn-offs" is extremely important. A woman moving from desire to arousal could be the difference between her partner smelling clean and fresh or him whispering sweet nothings or something sexual in her ear. We all have our list of things that drive us wild and they are so unique to each person.

In the book, *Come As You Are*, by Emily Nagoski, Ph.D (2015), she calls them "accelerators" and "brakes," and I love this description because that is exactly what they are. You are either moving further into the response cycle or *errrrrrrchh*, things can come to a complete stop. This abrupt halt can happen because of something so simple such as a tone of voice, a certain phrase that was spoken, or the presence of stinky sweaty bits. Whatever you choose to call them, your partner needs to know what turns you on and what turns you off and you, in turn, need to be well-versed in theirs. Communication is the key. When your partner knows what it takes to get you excited, they have such a huge advantage.

Just to make the point here let's visualize you and your partner trying to turn each other on. Let's say one of your turn-ons is having your hair gently played with and soft kisses on your neck. If your hubby comes in hot and starts aggressively playing with your hair and kissing your neck, it might not get you to where you need to be. If he knew that a slight adjustment would make the world of difference, don't you think he would tweak his moves in order to turn you on? Pretty sure he would be totally on board with this.

Shifting from the brake to the accelerator can be something so little but it can make a world of difference. I know that there is a long list of songs that when they start to play, my brain goes straight to sexy mode but if others were played, I'm out or I'll need a moment to redirect my energy. They are so specific to each person and if they are not shared and conveyed to your partner, he or she is coming into the game with a very clear disadvantage. Having a conversation about each other's lists could even be made into a fun little game. To get the convo started, I have included a fill-in-the-blank questionnaire to address this very topic in your workbook. If you can take a few minutes, I'm predicting that it may get really interesting and turn into a longer chat and that would be fantastic too. Take your time and write down everything that comes to mind that gets you going and then come back together and compare notes. I can almost guarantee you will learn something new or will be reminded of something that you had forgotten about what your partner loves. Check it out in your workbook, have fun with it, and it will prove to be one of the tools in your sexual toolbox that you will keep coming back to.

The differences between men and women, I find so compelling. When our differences are brought to the table and we are able to talk about them, we can then begin to understand each other a whole lot easier. Some things that we may not have understood before begin to make a whole lot more sense. Here is another difference that is incredibly interesting. When men want to show love to their partner and when they want to feel a deeper connection, their desire to have sex increases. On the flip side, when women feel loved and feel connected, their desire for sex increases. Do you see the potential issue here? Men have sex to feel loved, women want to feel loved in order to have sex. Men have sex to feel connected to their partner, women want and need to feel connected in order to want to be intimate with their spouse or partner and have sex.

Men → Sex = Love

Women → Love = Sex

Let's discuss a few more of the dissimilarities with sex, more specifically, in the orgasm department. With men, the orgasm is their pleasure point, and their main goal to achieve, but with women, it is the build-up, the excitement leading up to her release that drives them into untamed territory. A woman's climax has more variables to consider and is not quite as predictable as with men. A woman needs to be mindful and allow herself to let go of the multitasking that she has patterned herself to do. She needs to focus on the moment and how she is feeling and what she is feeling. She needs to embrace her sexuality, release her inner chatter, and just surrender in the moment. When she allows herself to do this, she can orgasm multiple times. Depending on the male's refractory period, he might be limited to one or he may be able to come back after a short period and be ready to go again.

So, as you can see, there are so many differences between men and women. Once they are out in the open and understood, things make more sense and we are able to get on the same page a whole lot quicker. When we choose to communicate and discuss these differences and how they affect us, our level of intimacy grows and the satisfaction level in the sex life department increases. When we are more informed, we can use this information going forward to make things work for us, not against us.

"Vulnerability- It is a skill that when purposefully practiced becomes one of the most useful and important tools in your relationship toolbox."

Shauna Harris

Chapter 9

Stay Curious

The one thing that we can always count on in life is change. Change is never ending, ongoing, and something that we shouldn't fear but instead, embrace. You are not the same person you were when you and your partner first met. You are not the same person as you were last year or yesterday. For that matter, twenty-four hours have past and we have each gone through a whole new set of experiences. For couples who say they know everything about their spouse, I disagree wholeheartedly. I guarantee that there are things that you do not know and have yet to discover. How can two different people from two totally different childhoods and upbringings think the same, feel the same and make the same decisions on a daily basis? You both probably have different careers and different personal goals. They can't be identical down to the letter, so there are always questions to ask and nooks and crannies to check out and explore.

Because life is always moving and constantly in motion, there are times and there will be times in your relationship where life gets in the way. Feelings of disconnect begin to creep in and something feels "off" or something just doesn't feel right. It is in these times that we need some quick fixes to try and reconnect. I have included a list of connecting questions for you to include in your relationship/sexuality toolbox. My hope here is for you to be able to use it as a tool to get the conversation started again. The purpose of these questions is meant to get the two of you engaged in a conversation and have fun while doing so. When you pick a question, each partner should answer the same question. You do not need to run through these questions like a speed dating session. You can choose just one or maybe a couple at a time. If I may suggest one thing, please just don't go through the list in one night. These are meant to start a meaningful conversations and bring the two of you closer.

1. What do you remember about the first day we met?
2. Do you remember what we did on our first date?
3. What do you remember about our first kiss?
4. What is your favorite date that we have ever gone on?
5. What did you think sex would be like with me?
6. What is one of your favorite intimate memories of us?
7. What is one of your favorite memories of us that was outside the bedroom?
8. What does sex mean to you?
9. What is your favorite out-of-the-bedroom kind of touch?
10. How often do you think about sex?
11. How many times would you ideally like to have sex/week?
12. What three things do you think that I like the best when we are between the sheets?

13. What three things do you like best in the bedroom?
14. Where are your favorite places to be touched or kissed between the sheets?
15. What was your favorite part about our wedding?
16. What is your favorite sexual position?
17. What was your favorite part about our honeymoon?
18. If you could travel anywhere in the world with me, where would we go?
19. Where would you most like to have sex that we never have before?
20. If I could do only one thing to you sexually, what would it be?
21. What new position would you be open to try?
22. What are your favorite things that I say during sex?
23. What is the easiest way to turn you on?
24. What song(s) puts you in the mood?
25. What is your least favorite position?
26. What is one positive change that you would make in our relationship?
27. Do you remember the first time you told me that you loved me?
28. What three qualities about me were you most attracted to?
29. What does being romantic mean to you?
30. What do I do outside of the bedroom that makes you want to get between the sheets?
31. What body part of yours is your favorite?
32. What body part of mine is your favorite?

33. What do I do that you think is sexy?

34. What would be your favorite romantic meal?

35. What are three things that I do for you that you are grateful for?

36. What is one thing that you would like to change about yourself?

37. What is one thing that I could more of for you outside of the bedroom?

38. What sex toy are you intrigues about or would you be willing to try?

39. What is a need that I could meet of yours right now or in the near future?

40. Who gave you the "birds & the bees" chat? How old were you?

41. What would be the funniest thing that could happen to us during sex?

42. What is your favorite way that I initiate sex?

43. If our house was on fire, what three things would you grab?

44. If your friends were asked to describe you, what would they say?

45. When did you first know you loved me?

46. What do you think our strengths are as a team?

47. What do I do that makes you feel loved?

48. What weird little thing(s) do I do that makes you shake your head but you really do like?

49. When was the last time you cried and why?

50. What is your favorite childhood memory?

51. What are the top five items on your "Bucket List?"

52. If you had a superpower, what would it be?

53. What was your favorite movie/book as a kid?

54. What three qualities do you admire about yourself?

55. What three qualities do you admire about me?

56. If you were given the opportunity to start any business, what would it be?

57. What is the most adventurous thing that you have ever done?

58. What is the most adventurous thing you think we have ever done?

59. How do you think you have changed over the last five years?

60. Where do you see us in five years? Ten years?

Well, there are a few questions to keep you going for a while but the list of things that you could ask your partner is endless. If you read the list or at least a few questions, you may have noticed that these questions go a little deeper than about *how* your partner is. Asking *how* your partner is can result in a one word answer and when you are trying to connect, a one-word answer just isn't going to get you into a deep conversation. You need to ask connecting questions. You want to know more about *who* your partner is.

Having meaningful conversations helps us feel more connected and stay connected. When we feel more connected to our partner, we feel more understood and the level of trust and the feeling of safety between partners increases. Now that we have come to understand what happens with our level of intimacy when the climate of our relationship is secure, we can take action steps to make some changes. When we begin to make small changes, action in the bedroom becomes more desired, sex becomes more frequently discussed and more consistently engaged in! In a nutshell, never stop asking your partner or your spouse questions! When we show interest in our loved one, it opens the doors of vulnerability, compassion, and creates a stronger bond. Never stop being inquisitive—stay curious, stay interested in each other's lives. This is such an important tool to put in your relationship toolbox. It shows your partner that they are important, that they matter to you, and that what they have to say holds value for you.

"It's not just about sex. Don't get me wrong, sex is great but when you have a connection with someone, when you feel so strongly for someone, just a kiss is enough to make your knees weak. You just can't beat that."

Anonymous

Chapter 10

Sex Does What?

We are all sexual beings. If you can learn to work together intentionally as a couple, to keep the level of intimacy at a comfortable level that works for the both of you, your relationship can be foolproof. The bonus of creating a sizzling sex life is actually more than meets the eye. There are many health benefits that sex brings to our lives and our relationship that you may not have realized, which gives us even more incentive and motivation to get it on between the sheets. Neurotransmitters are activated when we are engaged in sexual activity positively impacting our brains and several organs in our bodies as well. Here are some of the benefits of sex for men and women:

- Decreases depression
- Decreases anxiety
- Increases the connection and intimacy between partners
- Provides pain relief
- Increases the strength of the immune system
- Lowers blood pressure
- Improves heart health
- Increases self-esteem

- Improves quality of sleep
- Reduces stress
- Increases libido
- Increases level of intimacy
- Increases blood flow
- Improves complexion
- Improves bladder control (women)
- Relieves menstrual and premenstrual cramps (women)
- May lower prostate cancer risk (men)
- Reduces the chance of hypertension
- Reduces the chances of a stroke
- Strengthens muscles
- Burns calories
- Slows the aging process
- Makes babies
- It's fun

Now doesn't that list just increase the motivation and solidify the notion to have a little more sexy time with your spouse? Twenty-four amazing side effects to having sex with your partner and I didn't even go into detail. There is no prescription to fill, no magic pill. It doesn't cost you anything, your skin will glow and it will strengthen your relationship. What else on the planet does all of this? Nothing...let me repeat, nothing! And what is alarming is that studies show that adults between age eighteen and forty-four are engaging less and less frequently in sexual activity. There was an eighteen-year study done between 2000-2018 of over 9500 men and women. This research focused on the trends in the frequency of sexual activity. It was published in the *Journal of American Medical Association* (JAMA) in June 2020 and concluded that young people and married couples are having less sex.

- Nearly one in five (19%) women reported being sexually inactive between 2016-2018.

- More than one in five men (31%) reported being sexually inactive between 2016-2018.

- Between 2000 - 2002, 71% (married men) and 69% (married women) reported having sex weekly. In 2016-2018 those numbers decreased to 58% (married men) and 61% (married women) reportedly having sex weekly.

The reasons noted for the decrease in sex were attributed to an increase in people buying in to the daily grind and the busy schedules that we commit ourselves to; our fascination with technology and love for the screen; and an increase in mental health issues such as depression and anxiety. This disturbs me as an intimacy coach and as a sex educator because as I pointed out earlier, sex alleviates stress, anxiety, depression; it increases your confidence and releases feel good hormones. *Keep having sex! Make time for sex!* I cannot say this enough. It changes your relationship for the better and it makes you a healthier individual inside and out.

So many people rely on communicating through their phones instead of having a face-to-face conversation and our communication skills are suffering. What happens when our communication skills suffer? It highly affects our level of intimacy and when our level of intimacy begins to wane, our relationship suffers. Don't let the distractions of the world permeate the foundation of your relationship. Sometimes this is easier said than done but, if you notice this beginning to happen, check yourself. Be aware and make the necessary and much needed adjustments. Reach out to your partner, share how you are feeling and what you need, and connect. Create the kind of sex life that works for you and your partner and it will enhance your connection, your overall well-being, your physical and your mental health.

"The more I see you, the more I talk to you, the more I want you."

Unknown Author

Chapter 11

Initiating Sex

Everyone loves to be desired and loves to be the source or the reason that their partner is turned on. When important conversations have not been addressed and a common ground has not been paved, miscommunication and/or signals are bound to get crossed. If your partner comes on to you and you completely miss it or it comes across so subtly that you aren't really sure what they are communicating, it is time to make things clear. So many times what I used to think was a super clear and over-the-top obvious sign that I was interested in sex was not at all taken the same way by my hubby. I would feel a little bit frustrated and rejected and then think twice the next time I felt like doing it again. We finally had a conversation about it and ended up laughing so hard. He had absolutely no clue that what I had said at the time was my attempt to open the door to get it on.

It may seem silly to you that a discussion like this needs to happen but it does and let me tell you, it will make a world of difference in your relationship. Unclear messages cause hurt feelings, rejection, frustration, confusion, second-guessing, etc., when the message was not understood loud and clear. It's time to have a conversation about your top five moves that signal to your partner that you are in the mood for sex. Your partner then needs to do the same with you. Sometimes we think we are being so clear when in fact, our partner hears something completely different. We are left feeling unwanted and rejected and completely disconnected. This doesn't have to happen and it won't happen, if you effectively communicate.

Rejection is felt in the brain, the same place physical pain is felt so when someone is rejected, they feel real pain. Rejection hurts and when you are rejected time and time again, it can lead to resentment and angry feelings. We definitely don't want this, especially when it is an easy thing to avoid altogether. When we go into the situation with a vivid understanding about what candles beside the bed mean or a whisper in her ear or, "Hey honey, how about some sugar?", there will be no room for ambiguity. I hear a lot of my women clients say that their attempts at initiating sex are often ignored or dismissed and so they just give up. When I ask them to describe to me their initiating techniques and their best moves, their partner is so surprised and dumbfounded. They had no idea that what was conveyed was her interest in having sex and that she was looking for him to take the bait.

Once both sides are clear, there typically is a lot more sex happening because intentions are understood. There is no room for misinterpretation or a misunderstanding. This sounds so simple but it works. Communication is the key to a crazy amazing sex life and although this is just one very small piece, it makes for some very big results. Give it a shot. Get out a pen, open up your workbook, and start writing your top ways to initiate. I have provided two separate worksheets for you to each write in your favorites. You could even make it more interesting when you have each finished by letting your partner choose his or her favorites that you have written on your list.

Here is a little cheat sheet, if you need a teeny nudge to get your creative juices flowing. I have included a few ideas to get you started on your worksheets in your workbook. Your favorites might just be listed below or you may have totally different ones. It is ready for your input. Let's get some clarity on the page so we can start talking about initiating and clocking some more time between the sheets.

Some potential ideas for you:

- Whisper an "I want you" in their ear
- Send a naughty text
- Leave a VM
- Send a suggestive pic
- Leave a love note for them to find
- Give him/her a massage
- Run a bath
- Make their favorite dinner
- Drop an obvious hint
- Do their laundry
- Use humor
- Go to an adult sex shop
- Put up a "Post It" note
- Wear his/her favorite sexy outfit
- Set up a mini scavenger hunt with you as the prize
- Join them in the shower
- Light candles in the bedroom

- Subtle touches
- Go in for a make out session
- Get naked
- Be direct and just ask for it
- Help with the "To Do List"
- Leave a trail of clothes to the bedroom
- Gently play with their hair

Ask him/her what they would plan to do with you if you were naked right now

As I mentioned, these are just a few ideas. Everyone has their own unique ways to send the message that they would like to be intimate with their partner. Clarity in your actions and your overall communication is what is important here. For your partner to fully understand and for there to be no miscommunication in the initiating department, will be such a huge accomplishment. When you no longer have to deal with hurt feelings, feelings of rejection, or feelings of unworthiness it is a huge win for both parties. Who doesn't want that? And all it takes to get to this point is effective communication. You have the tools. You've got this! Make it a fun and lighthearted conversation. The feelings of connection and closeness that come with understanding one another on a deeper level are so rewarding and fulfilling so get let's start communicating!

"Challenges are what make life interesting; overcoming them is what makes life meaningful."

Joshua J Marine

Chapter 12

Seven-Day Challenge

Most things start with a decision. The first step in turning your sex life into a passionate, sparks flying, lip biting, toe curling, craving each other type of deal is just to decide that is the direction your relationship is going. Every interaction going forward takes you closer to that goal or farther away. It's on you and your partner to make it happen. Instead of running in a hamster wheel or feeling like it's Groundhog Day, day after day, it is time to put the brakes on the mundane train and make some small changes that add up to huge results.

Let's take a look at where you are and where you would like to be. There is a little bit of work that needs to be done before you reach your goal so take a look back at all of the things that you and your partner have tried. What has progressed you along the way and what has set you back? If there are some patterns that need to be broken, those areas are ones to be laser focused on. The more you practice, the easier it will become and the more habitual this behavior will be. Creating new and healthy ways to turn toward your partner and instill new healthy ways to respond when you are triggered will resolve conflicts along the way and will increase the level of intimacy in your relationship.

I have heard of, read about, and am well aware of a number of challenges, many of which have incorporated sexual activity in every day of the challenge. The challenges lasted anywhere from three to thirty days. I would like to do something a little bit different in this challenge. I highly encourage you to get between the sheets every day of this challenge, if that is what you feel so inclined to do but the goal for this challenge is to get you talking about sex and becoming more comfortable engaging in conversations about all things "sex."

Couples who talk about sex have higher levels of sexual satisfaction in their relationship so that is the main purpose for this challenge! There are a few guidelines when talking about sex with your partner, at any point in your relationship. I want to point these out to give you a leg up to help set you and your partner up for the best convos about sex. For this particular challenge, these guidelines are relevant but due to the nature and the purpose of this challenge, they aren't as much of a prerequisite because you know the conversations are coming.

You don't ever want to blindside or surprise your partner by a question having to do with your sex life, so timing is important. If you are reading this book together, there will not be any surprises this week but if you are reading this on your own, just give your spouse or partner a little notice to get in the right frame of mind. The suggestions that follow are not to make things more difficult. On the contrary, they are designed to help facilitate the conversations and help to bring a higher level of comfort and less awkwardness to your relationship. Here are the guidelines:

1. **Timing makes a difference.** It might not be a good time to bring on a convo about your sex life when your spouse is in the middle of a

workout or watching a basketball game. You know when your partner is preoccupied and is "knees deep" into an activity, this may not be the most appropriate time for a chat about the level of intimacy in your relationship. I also want to make a note that right after having sex with your partner is not the best time to talk about an issue or a problem that you may be experiencing in your sex life and wanting to change either.

2. **Pick a place**. I highly suggest to my clients to take the sex chats *out* of the bedroom. Keep them in a more neutral location. This makes the energy of the conversation more relaxed and open and not sexually charged — this is what the bedroom is for. There is no need to bring conversations about working on and bettering your sex life into the bedroom. This is where the magic happens. Keep it that way. When you designate your talks about sex to a more neutral location, it honestly makes it easier and more comfortable to discuss. Some of my clients like to have these discussions while on a walk together because it is easier to talk about sex initially if they don't have to maintain eye contact the entire time. When talking about sex is not yet a regular topic, this helps to alleviate awkward moments. You could even go for a drive, chat on the couch or in the backyard; wherever it is that makes you the least uncomfortable is where your place should be to chat.

3. **Give them a heads up**. When you are interested in talking about an issue that pertains to your sex life, set it up. Let your partner know

that you would love to talk about it and that way, they will be prepared to come to the table to talk about sex. You have had some time and have been thinking about it so it is respectful to provide them a little bit of time to do the same.

4. **Have a goal in mind**. Go into the chat with the goal to walk away feeling more connected and having come up with ways to work together.

5. Realize that **this will be an ongoing conversation** that will soon become a normal part of your relationship. This is not a one-time deal. These convos do not need to be long and drawn out if you are not into long conversations. They do not need to be short teeny discussions either. Make them work for you as a couple. There are no rules set in stone. Everyone has different needs and therefore everyone will have something different that works for them. The point here is just get talking about sex and then talking again, and then again, and again.

A seven-day challenge could be just what you need to give you a kickstart and show you that with intention and teamwork, some real changes can and will happen. If we start one day at a time for just seven days-just seven days-where could your relationship or marriage be? If we then can turn that one week into two weeks? Thirty days? Sixty days? Ninety days? Think about where it could be in such a short period of time if you just decide, commit, and get chatting. Patterns are challenging but never impossible to break. It's always easier when you have your best friend by your side, with some fun things to try, and some potential sex on the table. Who is with me?

Challenge Breakdown:

Day 1 — Now to Wow

Day 2 — Fail to Plan, Plan to Fail

Day 3 — Your Turn/My Turn

Day 4 — What If

Day 5 — Position Yourself

Day 6 — It's *Date Night*

Day 7 — Let's Make it Real

This challenge is going to be super simple and fun too. It is a challenge but it is not challenging by any means. It has been designed as a series of activities to complete together, as a couple, that is different than what you may have tried or done in the past. These activities can take as long as you want them to. There is no pressure. All I ask is that you try. Make an effort to commit to the seven days and see how much small efforts every day can add up to big changes. The worksheets that I mention for each day of the challenge can be found for your use, in the workbook that has been provided.

Day 1 — On the first day of this challenge your task is to look at where your relationship is right now and start a conversation about where you both want your sex life to be. Keep the conversation positive and upbeat. There are productive ways to achieve a "wow" sex life and pointing fingers isn't one of them. The purpose of this week is to take your sex dialogue game up a few notches. It is to start the conversation, if it hasn't happened, and make the topic of sex less awkward and a more regular guest at the conversation table. Set a goal that you both want to achieve together and a date by which you would like to achieve it. Fill out the sheet in your workbook together and commit to having some fun in the next seven days because these next seven days, if you are open to it, will change the way that you talk about sex from now on

Day 2 — When you make a plan, you set yourselves up to succeed. When you set a goal and have no direction in mind as to how on earth you are planning to get there, you are really planning to fail. A goal with a plan is a heck of a lot easier to reach because you know which steps to take to get to the desired result. So, on Day 2 let's talk about the frequency of sex that we desire each week or each month. Is it 2x a month? Is it 2x a week? Is it 4x a week? Talk about it. What would work for the both of you? If the number is different between the two of you then meet in the middle. Don't stress about the number, it isn't written in stone; it can be re-evaluated and changed. This has to work for both of you. You can even pick days that might work for you too. Many of my clients love to schedule their sexy time because then there is less chance of someone forgetting or of letting the days go by. This helps the low desire partner prepare for it and it helps the high desire partner because they are reassured that they will be getting their time between the sheets. Hop into your workbook and start making a plan!

Day 3 — Today is all about initiating. As previously talked about, initiating needs to come from both sides. One person should not be responsible for making all of the attempts to get the other between the sheets. You need to be fair and share half of the responsibility. So, if your number is 2x per week then one of you initiates one time and the other initiates the second time. Talk about your favorite ways to initiate and the favorite ways that your partner comes on to you. Take a peek at your "My Favorite Ways to Initiate" that you filled out from Chapter Eleven to refresh your memory, if needed. There is a worksheet in your workbook for you to take your discussion one step further about initiating. As we have previously learned, if you can better understand the ways in which your partner uses to send you the, "Let's get it on" message, it leaves much less room for miscommunication and rejection.

Day 4 — Today is a day to be creative and to think outside of the box. Today, we are going to include the phrase, "what if" to stir up your conversation about sex. I have included a page for each of you in your workbook to get you started. Let your imagination and your mind go here. Take a few minutes to fill out the questions. It won't take long, I promise. They are just little fire starters and the intention here is to learn something new about one another and to perhaps incorporate a few of these ideas in or out of the bedroom. There is no room for judgment here. The point is to start a conversation and enjoy each other's creativity and maybe spark an interest to try something new.

Day 5 — Today is all about trying new things! Is there a sex position that you have always wanted to try? Is there a position that you are curious about but have never brought it up with your spouse or partner? The conversation that is on the table today is stepping out of your routine and getting out of your comfort zone. Most couples rely on their go-to positions and usually their repertoire consists of between one to three different positions. When a couple engages in something new, the adrenaline in your body surges and the thrill of a new experience builds connection and bonding. My best advice here is to have fun and enjoy the experience. You can talk about what worked, what didn't work, what you liked, what you would like to change or try next time. Don't take things too seriously. If something feels weird or isn't feeling good, tweak it, get creative, and make it work for you. There are a few suggestions for today's challenge under Day 5 in your workbook. If you're feeling frisky or hot and bothered, tonight could be the night to try something new! You could even make an agreement that you pick one new position every couple of weeks or every month, whatever time frame seems best for the two of you.

Day 6 — We all know how important it is to spend quality time together and have fun together. Putting special time aside every week (strongly recommended) or every other week is so important to keep the connection strong and thriving in your relationship. Dates don't need to be elaborate nor even cost a lot of money at all. It is the effort made and the time spent together doing something fun or different that matters. I have included a list of dates earlier in the book for you in Chapter Seven, which provides a whole slew of ideas to choose from, or even be inspired by, to come up with your own. They range from staying home or close to home, to super adventurous, in hopes to appeal to everyone. If you find that you are stuck in a date rut and end up doing the same thing week after week, now is your chance to break the mold and try something new. Your relationship will thank you and you might even find a new favorite activity! Some of these ideas require some planning but a lot of them require minimal effort with maximum potential for enjoyment. Life is what you make of it so grab your partner and plan to have a great time together.

Go through the list and highlight the ones that you would like to engage in. You could even make more of a conversation piece out of it where each of you take a few minutes to grab a highlighter and pick out dates separately if you have not done that already. When you are both finished, you can chat about similar choices and different ones too. I challenge you to pick three to plan in the next three weeks: one from your list, one from your partner's list, and one that you both chose. *Never stop dating your spouse!* It is such an important part in making your relationship strong and thriving. Is it the date itself? Of course not. It is all about what the date generates and fosters in your marriage and in your relationship. Please feel free to utilize the worksheet provided in your workbook to write down three of your favorite new date ideas to try in the near future. If there are more ideas that pique your interest, write those down too. Even having your top five would be great to keep in mind for the next month or two.

Day 7 — Today is a day to look back at your week and see how the small intentional efforts made a difference in the level of intimacy between you and your partner. I have included a brief questionnaire to promote a convo about your individual thoughts and your collective thoughts on the activities that you have been a part of during this past week. What are a few things that you would like to incorporate into your weekly or monthly routine? Check out Day 7 in your workbook for today's summary questions. Remember, making a plan and committing to it is setting your sex life up for a much higher level of satisfaction. You can use the questions to start your conversation and come up with some more on your own, if you would like.

Every couple is unique in their own way, and everyone's situation is very different. There is not one "right" way to create your ideal relationship but the common thread that intertwines every couple that makes it long term is *connection* and *communication*. If you can make small, intentional efforts that turn into intentional daily habits, the level of intimacy and your sex live will be transformed. Taking the anxiety out of talking about sex can be such a big weight off your mind and your shoulders and if you can work towards this goal, the satisfaction in your sex life will skyrocket.

The more you talk about it, the easier it gets. Just like the saying, "practice makes perfect," although perfect is a figment of our imagination. But you get where I am going here. The more you talk about it, the easier it gets. I am a walking, breathing testament to this statement for sure and many of my clients are as well. There is such an straightforward, simple approach...just make it happen. Just put in the work and start talking. Is it always easy? Heck no! Is it a quick fix? No, not always, but it is a proven remedy and it is essential for long term success in any relationship.

Why is it so hard? Because we haven't been given the tools and we get wrapped up in the day-to-day patterns that have been ingrained in our minds. We assume or think that there are no concrete ways to fix certain situations that we find ourselves in when in fact, there totally is a better way. You just may need to look in a different direction for the answer or reach out and ask for some guidance and some assistance. You don't need to stay in a state of frustration or overwhelm. Your current situation can and will get better if you made the decision to do something about it.

Hand in hand,
You and me.
Today,
Tomorrow,
Forever.

~Anonymous

Conclusion

When you peel back the many layers of your relationship and look at what is at the core or the very foundation of what the two of you are made of, it is connection. If that connection begins to erode or is not tended to, the rest of the layers have nothing to build on.

I have been able to use what I have learned in my first marriage, what I have learned and am still learning in my second marriage, along with my years of training and experience of coaching couples, to re-create and help to build the connection that couples desire and long for. It may seem daunting and so out of reach but when it is broken down to the basics, it is not a complicated process at all.

Hoping for things to get better is fine but where does it get you? It gets you still hoping for things to get better years later. It takes you actually making a decision, committing to it with intention, using the action steps, and utilizing the tools provided to make some pretty incredible and long-lasting changes. Consistency will pay off big time in reaching for and achieving your sexuality goals when you make your relationship and your sex life a priority. If we spent as much time on nurturing our marriage as we do on our kiddos and our careers, life would look very different. Happy and successful relationships do not happen by pulling the long straw, or by chance. They just don't. We don't just deliver a baby and leave it to fend for itself; we take extra special care to ensure that it has everything that it needs and more. We have to start to look at our marriages a little bit more like this. When it needs to be taken care of, we can't put it on the back burner anymore. We have to address it with love and attention. When a problem arises it needs to be tended to and worked through until a solution is found.

> *The healthier your relationship is, the more fulfilling it will be.*

> *The healthier your sexual relationship is the more fulfilling it will be.*

> *The more positive things that you look for and acknowledge in your partner, the more positive things that you will see.*

> *The more positive things that you choose to see, the more positivity that you will see.*

When you make a commitment to be in a long-term relationship with someone, you are making the decision to do what it takes to succeed. It is like anything that you want to excel in, you have to put in the work. Your bank account isn't going to grow in numbers if you don't regularly make deposits. The same principle applies with your marriage or relationship. If you want it to be amazing, you need to make it amazing. It won't just happen. Your sex life won't just be off the charts, unless you raise the bar, make a decision, and stick to what it takes to make it reach new heights. It doesn't even require a massive amount of work but it does require small acts on a habitual and consistent basis. Regular and intentional small efforts add up to big changes and strong foundations that will set you and your spouse or partner up for the most amazing and fulfilling sex life and relationship as a whole.

If you have not yet set a goal for yourself and your relationship, it's time for you to step up to the plate, right here right now! Make a decision to improve your sex life and watch how your life will begin to change in all areas. You need to build habits that serve you and your marriage and remove those that are holding you back from enjoying yourself and your partner to the fullest.

I mentioned before that making a plan is a surefire way to get you on your way to fulfilling your sexuality goals. When you have a vision, and then you have a plan, there is a clear path of where you need and desire to go. If you are a little stumped as to how to create a plan, I will give you the steps to help guide you. Think about what your goal looks like. What does your relationship and your sex life look like in your wildest dreams? Do you want to be able to freely ask for what you want and need in the bedroom? Do you want to be able to feel so comfortable and confident in your sexuality that you can let go of your insecurities and just be in the moment? Do you want to be able to suggest new positions without second guessing yourself or feeling scared that you will be judged or rejected? Whatever your ideal sex life looks like, you can achieve it with a plan.

1. What is your goal? Be specific and focus on what you really want. What it is you want intrinsically?

2. What is the outcome that you are after? What does your finish line look like to you? This way you can be results-driven and have a clear vision in mind that will keep you motivated and on track.

3. What is your why? What is the reason behind the need for this goal to be achieved? You are more likely to achieve your goal when there is a personal meaning attached to it for you.

4. Be vulnerable. In order to reach this goal you are going to have to be prepared to be open, honest, and vulnerable. This might be challenging at first for you but it is one of the more important steps in achieving the sex life that you are working towards.

5. Set small reachable goals. Set yourself and your partner up for success and make small attainable goals that ultimately achieve your goal. You could even set a date as to when you would like to be in the spicy zone with your partner or spouse.

6. Celebrate the wins along the way! If there is progress made and the finish line is getting closer, honor, recognize, and acknowledge the work and effort that you have put in. A win is a win, progress is progress and it needs to be acknowledged!

Be realistic. This will not happen overnight. It took you awhile to get where you are so it is going to take some time to get you where you want to be. The plans that I help my clients create are usually sixty or ninety day plans. This way the pressure is taken off. It is also important to make the process fun and enjoyable so that you both are excited to move forward together. Be intentional. You have made a decision to better your relationship, so do it. And please, don't forget to praise each other for the wins, big or small. I cannot stress this enough, progress needs to be commended with teeny or monstrous celebrations. We are more prone to look forward and be motivated to continue on the path to achieving the goal when we are positively reinforced. Remember, when we focus on the positive in any situation, we tend to see more positive results.

The key to a successful relationship and a mind blowing sex life is the emotional connection that you decide to create and continue to make an effort to maintain. If you want to increase your sexual satisfaction, remember it doesn't start in the bedroom. You will most certainly reap the rewards, and then some, between the sheets but what you do and the efforts that you make to connect and to stay connected, will make a vast difference in the quality of your sex life. When you both utilize the tools and techniques that I have shared, you will begin to see things change. The more you make an effort to connect and practice the conflict resolution steps, the easier it gets. The stronger the foundation you build, the less crumbly your relationship will be when there is storm brewing.

When you are connected outside of the bedroom, it is 100 percent, hands down easier to then feel connected inside of the bedroom. One last piece of solid advice: Put the book down and start making the small efforts to touch and to communicate and to understand one another on a level that you have never been to before. In no time your sex life will be one to blush about and be proud of and you should be! Your marriage/your relationship is a beautiful masterpiece in the making that deserves the care and attention of your most cherished asset, because that is exactly what it is and should be!

"Love isn't always perfect.
It isn't a fairytale or a storybook.
And it doesn't always come easy.

Love is overcoming obstacles;
Facing challenges, fighting to be together,
Holding on & never letting go.
It is a short word, easy to spell,
Difficult to define, & impossible to live without.

Love is work, but most of all,
Love is realizing that every hour,
Every minute, & every second was worth it
Because you did it together."

Author Unknown

Thank you for going on this journey with me! If you would like to reach out and are interested in further guidance or working with me personally, I would be honored to help you take your relationship to the next level. I can be reached at shauna@exploreintimacy.com or https://www.exploreintimacy.com

I look forward to hearing from you.

References

Charoensukmongkol P. (2014) *Benefits of mindfulness meditation on emotional intelligence, general self-efficacy, and perceived stress: Evidence from Thailand*. Journal of Spirituality in Mental Health, 16(3), 171-192.

Goleman D. (1995). *Emotional intelligence: Why it can matter more than IQ.* New York, NY: Bantam Books.

Johnson, S. (2008). *Hold me tight*. New York, NY. Little Brown.

Nagoski, E. (2015). *Come as you are*. New York, NY: Simon & Schuster.

Tielemans, S. (2020). *Communications secrets master class* {Notes}

The Gottman Method. (2020). The Gottman Institute. Retrieved from https://www.gottman.com/about/the-gottman-method/

Zaccaro A., Piarulli A., Laurino M., Garbella, E., Menicucci, N., Gemignani A. (2018). *How breath-control can change your life: A systematic review on psycho-physiological correlates of slow breathing*. Front Hum Neurosci, 12, 353.

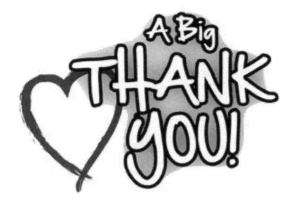

Thank You For Reading My Book!

CAN YOU HELP?

I really appreciate all of your feedback and I love hearing what you have to say.

I need your input to make the next version of this book and my future books better.

Please leave me a review on Amazon letting me know what you thought of the book.

Thanks so much!

Shauna Harris

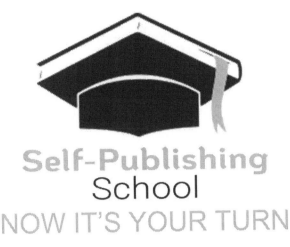

Self-Publishing School
NOW IT'S YOUR TURN

Discover the EXACT 3-step blueprint you need to become a bestselling author in as little as 3 months.

Self-Publishing School helped me, and now I want them to help you with this FREE resource to begin outlining your book!

Even if you're busy, bad at writing, or don't know where to start, you CAN write a bestseller and build your best life.

With tools and experience across a variety of niches and professions, Self-Publishing School is the <u>only</u> resource you need to take your book to the finish line!

DON'T WAIT

Say "YES" to becoming a bestseller:

https://self-publishingschool.com/friend/

Follow the steps on the page to get a FREE resource to get started on your book and unlock a discount to get started with Self-Publishing School.

Made in the USA
Middletown, DE
09 January 2024